NURSING PHOTOBOOK™

Performing GI Procedures

NURSING82 BOOKS
INTERMED COMMUNICATIONS, INC.
SPRINGHOUSE, PENNSYLVANIA

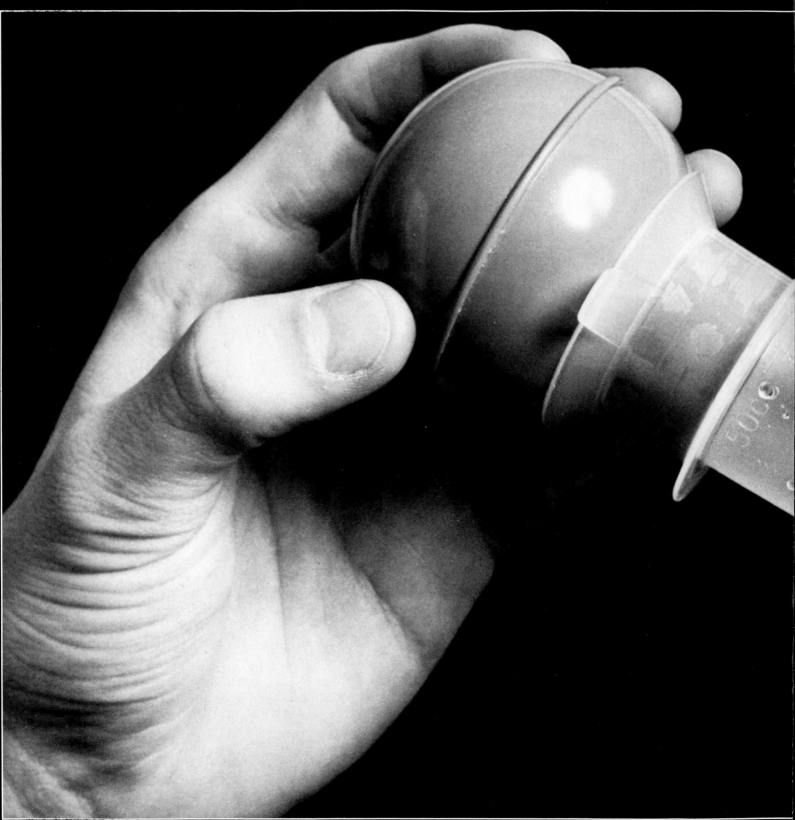

Performing GI Procedures

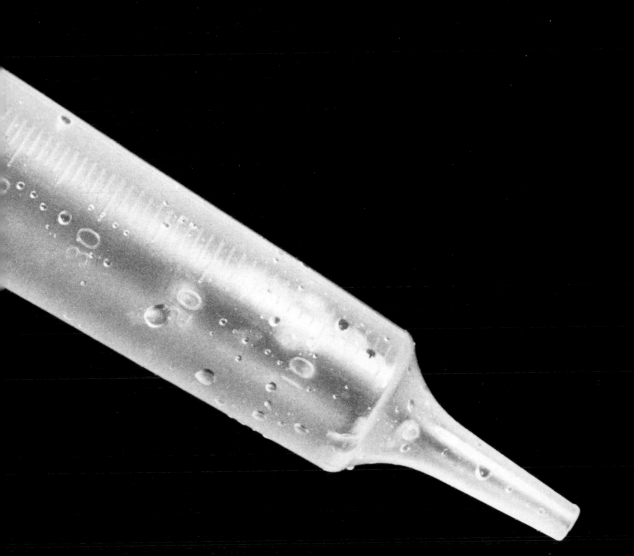

NURSING82 BOOKS

NURSING PHOTOBOOK™ SERIES
Providing Respiratory Care
Managing I.V. Therapy
Dealing with Emergencies
Giving Medications
Assessing Your Patients
Using Monitors
Providing Early Mobility
Giving Cardiac Care
Performing GI Procedures
Implementing Urologic Procedures
Controlling Infection
Ensuring Intensive Care
Coping with Neurologic Disorders
Caring for Surgical Patients
Working with Orthopedic Patients
Nursing Pediatric Patients
Helping Geriatric Patients
Attending Ob/Gyn Patients
Aiding Ambulatory Patients
Carrying Out Special Procedures

NURSING SKILLBOOK® SERIES
Reading EKGs Correctly
Dealing with Death and Dying
Managing Diabetics Properly
Assessing Vital Functions Accurately
Helping Cancer Patients Effectively
Giving Cardiovascular Drugs Safely
Giving Emergency Care Competently
Monitoring Fluid and Electrolytes Precisely
Documenting Patient Care Responsibly
Combatting Cardiovascular Diseases Skillfully
Coping with Neurologic Problems Proficiently
Using Crisis Intervention Wisely
Nursing Critically Ill Patients Confidently

NURSE'S REFERENCE LIBRARY™
Diseases
Diagnostics

Nursing82 **DRUG HANDBOOK™**

PROFESSIONAL GUIDE TO DRUGS™

NURSING PHOTOBOOK™ Series

PUBLISHER
Eugene W. Jackson

EDITORIAL DIRECTOR
Jean Robinson

CLINICAL DIRECTOR
Barbara McVan, RN

ART DIRECTOR
Lisa A. Gilde

Intermed Communications Book Division

DIRECTOR
Timothy B. King

DIRECTOR, RESEARCH
Elizabeth O'Brien

DIRECTOR, PRODUCTION AND PURCHASING
Bacil Guiley

Staff for this volume

BOOK EDITOR
Patricia Reilly Urosevich

CLINICAL EDITOR
Mary Horstman Obenrader, RN

ASSOCIATE EDITOR
Sally Nimaroff Sapega

PHOTOGRAPHER
Paul A. Cohen

DESIGNERS
Linda Jovinelly Franklin
Carol Stickles

ASSOCIATE PHOTOGRAPHER
Thomas Staudenmayer

EDITORIAL/GRAPHIC COORDINATOR
Doreen K. Stowers

CLINICAL/GRAPHIC COORDINATOR
Evelyn M. James

COPY EDITOR
Eric R. Rinehimer

EDITORIAL STAFF ASSISTANT
Cynthia A. O'Connell

PHOTOGRAPHY ASSISTANT
Frank Margeson

ART PRODUCTION MANAGER
Wilbur D. Davidson

ARTISTS
Darcy Feralio   Louise Stamper
Diane Fox   Joan Walsh
Robert Perry   Ron Yablon
Sandra Simms

TYPOGRAPHY MANAGER
David C. Kosten

TYPOGRAPHY ASSISTANTS
Janice Haber
Ethel Halle
Diane Paluba
Nancy Wirs

PRODUCTION MANAGERS
Robert L. Dean, Jr.
Kathy Murphy

ASSISTANT PRODUCTION MANAGER
Deborah C. Meiris

PRODUCTION ASSISTANT
Donald G. Knauss

ILLUSTRATORS
Jack Crane   Donald S. Johnson
Darcy Feralio   Kurt M. Loeb
Jean Gardner   Henry Rothman
Tom Herbert   Bud Yingling
Robert Jackson

SERIES GRAPHIC DESIGNER
John C. Isely

COVER PHOTO
Seymour Mednick

Clinical consultants for this volume

Marjorie L. Beck, RN
Charge Nurse, GI Procedure Unit
Abington Memorial Hospital
Abington, Pa.

Mary Jane Koch, RN, BA, ET
Medical Affairs Department Manager
Hollister, Incorporated
Chicago, Ill.

Copyright © 1982, 1981 by Intermed
Communications, Inc.,
1111 Bethlehem Pike, Springhouse, Pa. 19477
All rights reserved. Reproduction in
whole or part by any means
whatsoever without written permission
of the publisher is prohibited by law.
Printed in the United States of America
030682

Library of Congress Cataloging in Publication Data

Main entry under title:

Performing GI procedures.

 (Nursing81 books) (Nursing Photobook)
 Bibliography: p.
 Includes index.
 1. Gastrointestinal system—Diseases—Nursing—Pictorial
works. I. Series. II. Series: Nursing Photobook.
 [DNLM: 1. Gastroenterology—Methods—Nursing texts.
WY 156.5 P438]
RC802.P46   616.3'30754   81-965
ISBN 0-916730-31-X   AACR2

Contents

Contributors

At the time of original publication, these contributors held the following positions.

Marjorie L. Beck, an adviser for this PHOTOBOOK, is charge nurse for the GI procedure unit, Abington Memorial Hospital, Abington, Pa. She earned her nursing diploma from the Abington Memorial Hospital School of Nursing. She belongs to the American Nurses Association, the Pennsylvania Nurses Association, and the Society of Gastrointestinal Assistants.

Mike D'Orazio is director of enterostomal therapy at Albert Einstein Medical Center in Philadelphia. A graduate of St. Joseph's University in Philadelphia, and the Harrisburg (Pa.) Hospital Enterostomal Therapy School, he's a certified enterostomal therapist. In addition, Mr. D'Orazio is cofounder of Delaware Valley Enterostomal Therapists, adviser and member of the Philadelphia Ostomy Association and the Delaware County Ostomy Association. He also belongs to the International Association for Enterostomal Therapy.

Mary Jane Koch, also an adviser for this PHOTOBOOK, is medical affairs department manager, Hollister Incorporated, Chicago. She's also a Major in the United States Air Force Reserve Nursing Corps, 31st Air Evacuation Squad, Charleston Air Force Base, S.C. She received her nursing diploma from St. Vincent's Hospital and Medical Center, New York City, a BA from Jersey City (N.J.) State College, and she's a graduate of the Enterostomal Therapy Program, Boston University. Ms. Koch is a certified enterostomal therapist. Currently, she's an MA candidate at Loyola University, Chicago. In addition, she is a United States delegate to the World Council of Enterostomal Therapists, vice-president of the Nurse Consultants Association, and an associate fellow in the Aerospace Medical Association. She belongs to the American Nurses Association, National League of Nurses, Oncology Nurse Association, International Association of Enterostomal Therapists, Association of Rehabilitation Nurses, Association of Practitioners of Infection Control, American Urologic Association Allied, and the Reserve Officers Association.

Barbara K. Rideout is in-service coordinator, and a certified enterostomal therapist, at Graduate Hospital, Philadelphia. She earned her nursing diploma from the Sacred Heart School of Nursing, Allentown, Pa., and her BSN from the University of Delaware (Newark). She's a member of the Delaware Valley Enterostomal Therapists, and the International Association for Enterostomal Therapy.

Susan E. Sweny is GI nurse coordinator at Mount Auburn Hospital, Cambridge (Mass.). She's a graduate of the Mt. Auburn School of Nursing. Ms. Sweny is a member and past president of the Society of Gastrointestinal Assistants, and is an adviser to the Digestive Diseases Education and Information Clearinghouse.

Alicia Alphin-Tollison former assistant professor, University of Tennessee (Memphis) College of Nursing, received her BSN from the University of Tennessee College of Nursing, and her MN from Emory University in Atlanta.

Introduction

If you've ever changed a gastrostomy dressing, applied a disposable ostomy pouch, or administered a retention enema, you have performed a GI procedure. And regardless of where you work, GI procedures are part of your nursing responsibility. Unquestionably, then, you need to continually review and update your GI nursing skills.

So, we've written this NURSING PHOTOBOOK for you. In it, you'll find over 100 step-by-step GI procedures that take you past the basics. For example, do you know how to use a volumetric pump to administer a tube feeding? How to help the doctor insert a Sengstaken-Blakemore tube? Or how to manage a draining fistula? If not, we provide the answers. But that's not all we've included. You'll also learn how to obtain specimens for gastric analysis, how to assist the doctor with lower GI endoscopy, and how to perform an iced gastric lavage.

As you page through this PHOTOBOOK, you'll be amazed at the number of GI procedures we've covered. We show you how to cope with all types of esophagogastric, intestinal, gallbladder, hepatic, and pancreatic disorders. We tell you, as well as show you, how to care for a patient who's had a cholecystectomy or a gastric resection, and how to care for one who has hepatitis. And our informative illustrations will help refresh your memory on GI anatomy.

The most comprehensive portion of this PHOTOBOOK includes up-to-the-minute information on how to select, apply, and remove ostomy pouches, skin barriers, and adhesives. Our easy-to-read captions and clear, sharply focused photographs will guide you through a colostomy irrigation, including how to dilate your patient's stoma.

Are you teaching a patient how to empty his ostomy pouch or clean a reusable one? If so, be sure to give him a copy of one of the special home care aids we've included for your use.

Be looking for the eye-catching logos throughout this PHOTOBOOK. They alert you to valuable additional information on patient preparation and special situations.

All in all, this PHOTOBOOK promises to make you a more competent, knowledgeable member of the health care team. Then you can be confident you're giving the best care possible.

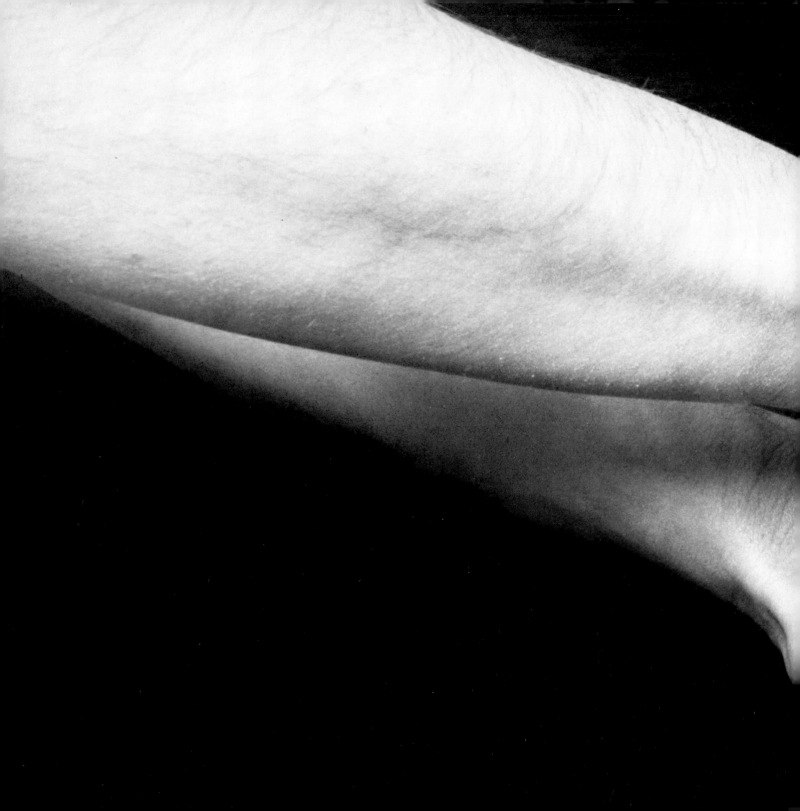

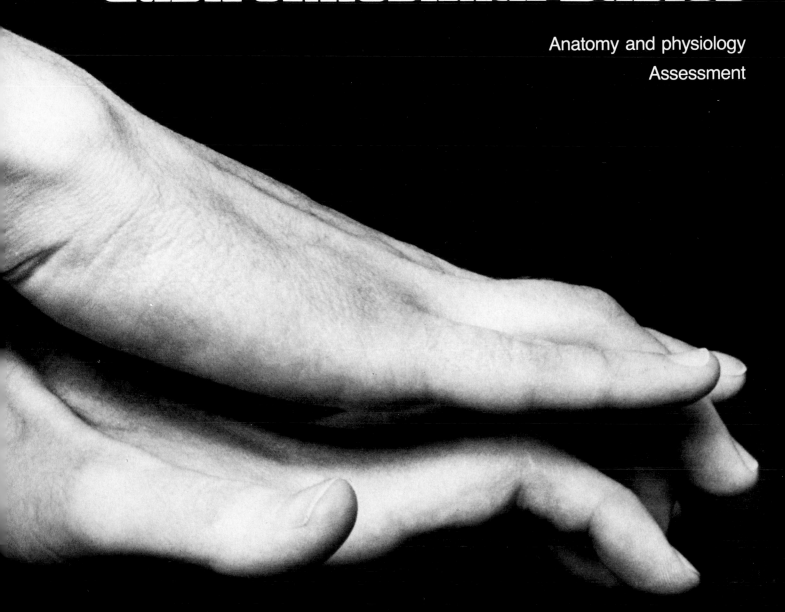

Understanding Gastrointestinal Basics

Anatomy and physiology

Assessment

Anatomy and physiology

How familiar are you with the gastrointestinal (GI) system? Before we discuss GI procedures, you'll want to learn how to assess a healthy GI tract. You'll also want to know the normal structure and function of each organ in the GI system. Test your knowledge of the fundamentals. Do you know:

• how to observe and assess your patient's abdomen?
• how to collect and evaluate GI data properly?
• which hormone inhibits gastric secretion?
• which organ produces bile?

On the next few pages we'll give you the answers to these questions and others. Read this section carefully.

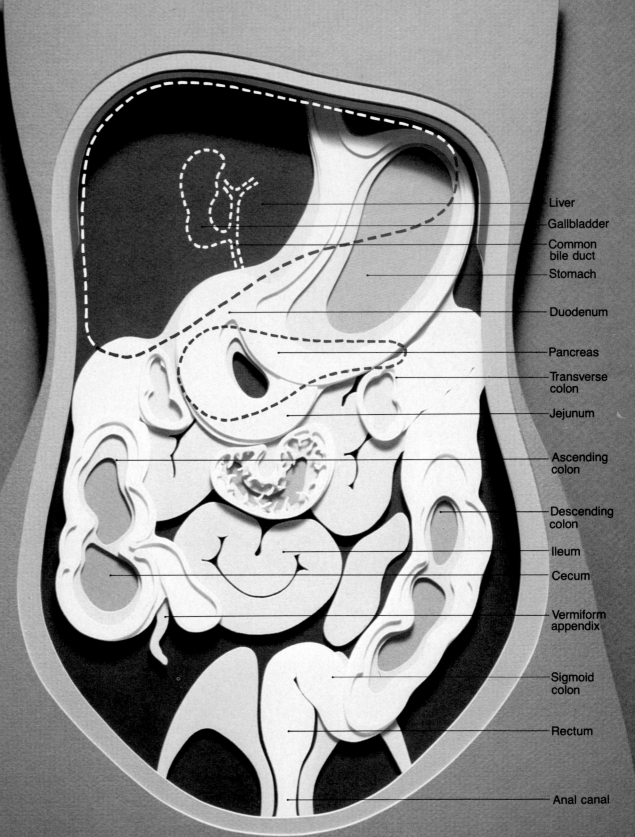

Liver
Gallbladder
Common bile duct
Stomach
Duodenum
Pancreas
Transverse colon
Jejunum
Ascending colon
Descending colon
Ileum
Cecum
Vermiform appendix
Sigmoid colon
Rectum
Anal canal

Recognizing GI structures

	Description	Digestive function
Mouth and throat 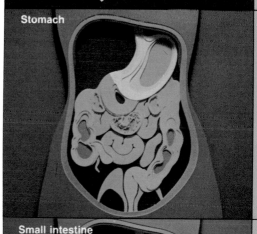 Tongue Mouth Pharynx Trachea Teeth	• Consists of lips, cheeks, teeth, tongue, palate, salivary glands, and pharynx • Initial portion of digestive tract	• Teeth break up food, increasing the total surface area of the food, which allows for more rapid and efficient digestion. • Salivary glands produce saliva, which contains mucus and an enzyme, ptyalin. Ptyalin breaks down starches, and mucus helps lubricate and moisten food. • Voluntary tongue movement causes food to move into pharynx; from there, food is carried into the esophagus by the involuntary second phase of swallowing.
Esophagus Esophagus	• Tubelike structure, about 10″ (25 cm) long, located behind trachea but in front of vertebral column • Connects mouth to stomach	• Secretes mucus, which facilitates swallowing and prevents reflux gastric juices from breaking down the esophageal wall. • Peristalsis and gravitational force move food through esophagus toward stomach.
Stomach	• Elongated pouchlike structure, located below diaphragm in upper abdomen • Approximately five sixths of stomach lies to left of the midline.	• Secretes gastric juices, which mix with food to form chyme. • Absorbs water, alcohol, and glucose from chyme. • Stores food before chyme enters small intestine. • Causes slow emptying of chyme into small intestine through peristalsis and contractions of the pylorus and duodenal bulb. The rate varies with volume and chemical composition of food.
Small intestine	• Tubelike structure about 18′ (5.5 m) long and 1″ (2.5 cm) in diameter. Extends from distal end of pyloric sphincter to ileocecal orifice, filling most of lower abdominal cavity • Divided into three parts: duodenum, jejunum, and ileum	• Chyme in duodenum stimulates release of hormones, which in turn activate enzymes from liver, gallbladder, pancreas, and duodenal mucosa. These enzymes break down fats, proteins, and carbohydrates. • Absorbs water and nutrients from chyme. • Peristalsis and segmentation move chyme through small intestine to large intestine.

Anatomy and physiology

Recognizing GI structures continued

	Description	Digestive function
Large intestine	• Tubelike structure about 6' (1.8 m) long and 2½" (6.3 cm) in diameter. Located in lower abdomen. • Consists of three parts: cecum (located in lower right abdomen); colon, which includes the vermiform appendix (outlines abdominal cavity and is divided into ascending, transverse, descending); and sigmoid colon (located on anterior surface of sacrum and coccyx) which includes anal canal and rectum.	• Absorbs water and salts from chyme. • Secretes mucus, which lubricates and protects intestinal lining. • Ileocecal valve allows slow passage of chyme to colon and prevents backflow to small intestine. • Eliminates digestive wastes. • Peristalsis and segmentation move chyme through colon to rectum and initiate urge to defecate.
Pancreas	• Lobulated structure about 9" (22.9 cm) long. Located behind stomach; the wide end connects to duodenum, narrow end touches spleen. • Pancreatic duct opens into duodenum	• Secretes pancreatic juice into duodenum. Pancreatic secretion's regulated by two intestinal hormones, secretin and pancreozymin. • Pancreatic juice contains enzymes that break down carbohydrates, fats, and protein; also, the juice contains bicarbonate ions, which help neutralize chyme.
Gallbladder	• Pear-shaped structure about 4" (10 cm) long. Located on liver's undersurface. • Connected to upper portion of duodenum by common bile duct.	• Concentrates bile. • Stores up to 50 ml of bile. • Chyme (particularly with large fat content) in duodenum causes release of hormone (cholecystokinin), which activates muscular contractions in gallbladder, pushing bile into duodenum.
Liver	• Large, brownish-red gland, located under diaphragm in upper portion of abdomen. • Largest organ in body; weighs about 3 pounds (1.4 kg) in an adult. • Connected to common bile duct by hepatic duct.	• Continuously produces bile, which is then stored in the gallbladder. • Stores glycogen, fat-soluble vitamins, and some water-soluble vitamins. • Metabolizes carbohydrates, fats, and proteins.

Learning about peristalsis

To get an idea of how peristalsis works, try squeezing a toothpaste tube with your hand. As your fingers press the sides of the tube together, the contents push forward, as shown in the illustration at top right. In peristalsis, a series of wavelike contractions continually pushes food from the pharynx to the rectum, along the GI tract.

What causes peristalsis? An accumulation of food in the GI tract (tube distention) triggers peristaltic contractions.

The peristaltic rate is amazingly adaptive, (see bottom-right illustration) decreasing and increasing according to the body's digestive and absorption needs. The first, or primary, peristaltic contraction begins in the pharynx. As you know, this contraction pushes food through the esophagus into the stomach, and takes about 5 to 10 seconds. Secondary peristalsis moves any remaining food into the stomach.

Unlike the quick primary peristaltic contraction, the stomach's peristalsis is much slower, averaging about three contractions per minute. However, during the journey from the small intestine to the large intestine, the peristaltic rate increases from 0.5 cm per second (in the top portion of the small intestine) to 5 cm per second (when the chyme reaches the large intestine).

The movement of chyme from the pylorus to the ileocecal valve takes about 3 to 10 hours. To allow absorption at this point, peristaltic contractions spread chyme along the intestinal wall.

Large-scale peristalsis begins in the colon. The strong—but brief (about 15 minutes)—burst of peristaltic contractions pushes the intestinal contents through the colon. These movements occur only a few times a day, usually after meals. The final push of fecal matter, from the colon into the rectum, is the last peristaltic contraction. This accumulation of fecal matter in the rectum triggers the urge to defecate.

Study these illustrations to better understand peristaltic contractions.

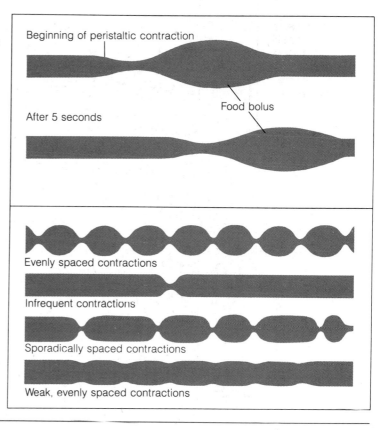

Beginning of peristaltic contraction

Food bolus

After 5 seconds

Evenly spaced contractions

Infrequent contractions

Sporadically spaced contractions

Weak, evenly spaced contractions

Understanding hormones and digestive juices

In the digestive process, hormones activate the digestive juices that break down foods. The more you know about the relationships between these hormones and digestive juices, the better you'll understand the gastrointestinal system. The chart below and the one on pages 14 and 15 explain, in detail, the function of each hormone and digestive juice in the digestive process.

Hormone	Source	Activating substances	Action
Gastrin	Gastric mucosa of the pylorus	• Partially digested proteins in pylorus	• Stimulates release of gastric juice
Enterogastrone	Mucosa of small intestine	• Fats, sugar, and acids in intestine	• Inhibits gastric secretion
Villikinin	Mucosa of small intestine	• Chyme in intestine	• Stimulates intestinal villi movements
Secretin	Duodenal mucosa	• Partially digested proteins, fats, and acids in intestine	• Stimulates pancreatic juice
Pancreozymin	Duodenal mucosa	• Partially digested proteins, fats, and acids in duodenum	• Stimulates pancreatic juice
Cholecystokinin	Duodenal mucosa	• Fats in duodenum	• Stimulates gallbladder contractions leading to release of bile

Anatomy and physiology

Nurses' guide to digestive juices

DIGESTIVE JUICE	SOURCE	PRINCIPLE ENZYME
Saliva	Salivary glands	Ptyalin (amylase)
Gastric juice	Stomach	Pepsin
		Gastric lipase
Bile	Liver (stored in and released from gallbladder)	None
Pancreatic juice	Pancreas	Trypsin
		Chymotrypsin
		Pancreatic lipase
		Pancreatic amylase
		Nucleases
		Carboxypeptidases
	Duodenal mucosa	Enterokinase
		Aminopeptidases
		Dipeptidase
		Sucrase
		Lactase
Intestinal juice	Intestinal villi	Maltase
		Nucleotidase
		Nucleosidase
		Intestinal lipase

WHAT IT ACTS ON	RESULTING PRODUCTS
Starch	Dextrins, maltose
Proteins	Polypeptides
Emulsified fats	Fatty acids, glycerol
Unemulsified fats	Emulsified fats
Denatured proteins, polypeptides	Polypeptides, amino acids
Proteins, polypeptides	Polypeptides, amino acids
Bile-emulsified fats	Fatty acids, glycerol
Starch	Maltose
Nucleic acids	Nucleotides
Polypeptides	Smaller polypeptides
Trypsinogen	Trypsin
Polypeptides	Smaller polypeptides
Dipeptides	Amino acids
Sucrose	Glucose, fructose
Lactose	Glucose, galactose
Maltose	Glucose
Nucleotides	Nucleosides, phosphoric acid
Nucleosides	Purine, pentose
Fat	Glycerides, fatty acids, glycerol

Assessment

Assessing your patient's GI system? If so, do you know how to inspect your patient's teeth? Or check his salivary glands?

Do you know how to check a patient for abdominal rebound tenderness? Can you tell if he has an obstructed bowel?

The next sequence will take you through a step-by-step gastrointestinal assessment. We'll explain how to gather baseline data, and give you some sample questions you may want to ask your patient. We've also included some valuable tips on evaluating the findings of your examination.

How to auscultate, percuss, and palpate

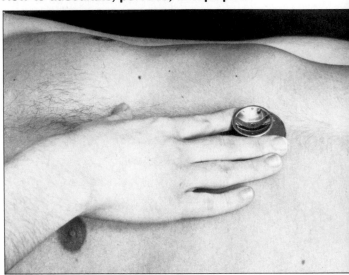

DOCUMENTING

Documenting gastrointestinal data

Before you assess your patient's GI system, you'll need pertinent information about his medical history, lifestyle, and family history. Obtain this data by observation, inspection, and interviewing. During the interview, you may want to ask your patient these questions:

• Do you have any problems chewing or swallowing food?
• Describe the condition of your teeth. When was your last dental exam? What did the doctor find? Did you have any cavities or infections? When was your last set of oral X-rays taken?
• Rate your sense of taste. Is it excellent? Good? Fair? Or poor? Are you able to distinguish flavors? Have you noticed any change in your ability to taste? Or any peculiarities?
• Do you have any loose or missing teeth? If so, which ones? How long have they been loose or missing?
• Do you wear dentures? If so, how long have you been wearing them? How do they fit? Do you use dental adhesive?
• How do your gums feel? Do they bleed? Do you have sores on your gums or tongue?
• Have you noticed any bleeding from your mouth? If so, when?
• How does your throat usually feel? When was your last sore throat? How many sore throats do you have yearly? Do you take anything to relieve them?
• Have you ever had a broken jaw or an injury to your mouth or teeth? If so, describe the details.
• Have you ever had any type of oral surgery? If so, describe the details.
• Have you had any pain in your stomach or abdomen? If so, can you describe it? How often do you feel the pain? Is it intermittent, or constant? Does anything relieve the pain or make it worse; for example, eating?
• Do you vomit frequently? If so, how frequently? Describe the vomitus. Have you ever vomited blood? Is your vomitus ever dark brown or black? Do you ever take any medication for vomiting? If so, what?
• How is your appetite?
• Have you ever been X-rayed for an ulcer? If so, when? Have you ever been treated for an ulcer? If so, when? Do you still have any pain from your ulcer?
• Have you ever had indigestion, heartburn, or gas? If so, does it usually occur after you eat certain foods? Do you take medication to relieve it? If so, what?
• How often do you have a bowel movement? Do you take laxatives? If so, how frequently? Do you have more than two loose stools a day? If so, do you take medication for this? What kind?
• Do you ever have blood in your stool? If so, how often? Is the blood mixed in with the stool or does it coat the surface?
• Do you ever have clay-colored stools?
• Do you ever have frothy stools?
• Are your stools ever pencil thin?
• Do your stools float? Do you ever have black stools?
• Have you ever had your colon X-rayed? If so, when? Have you ever undergone a colonoscopy or proctoscopy? If so, why? How long ago?
• Have you ever had abdominal surgery? If so, when? What type was it?
• Do you have a colostomy or an ileostomy? If so, how long have you had it? Why was it done? How do you care for it?
• When was the last time you went to a doctor for abdominal or intestinal problems?
• Do you have hemorrhoids?
• Can you describe any other problems?

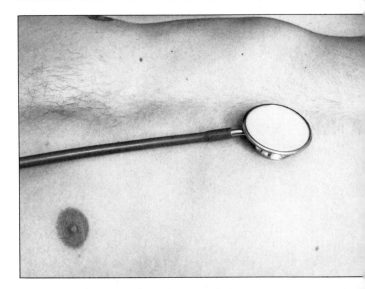

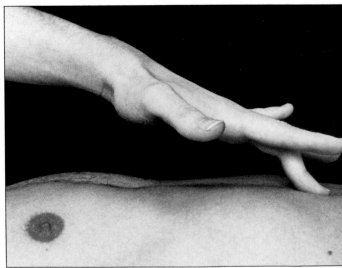

1 *Assessing your patient's GI system? If so, you'll use your skills of auscultation, percussion, and palpation. Always auscultate your patient's abdomen before you palpate or percuss it. Palpation and percussion may change the frequency of his peristaltic sounds.*

When you auscultate your patient, you'll use a stethoscope to assess the sounds produced by various arteries, organs, and tissues.

To assess high-frequency sounds, you'll use the diaphragm side of the stethoscope's chest piece. Always position the diaphragm's entire surface firmly on your patient's skin.

Note: To improve the diaphragm's contact and reduce extraneous noise, apply water or water-soluble jelly to your patient's skin before auscultating.

2 You'll use the stethoscope's bell to assess low-frequency sounds. To do this, *lightly* place the bell on your patient's skin. Be careful not to exert pressure on the bell. If you do, your patient's skin will act as a diaphragm, causing you to miss low-frequency sounds.

3 Next, percuss your patient's abdomen to determine the density, size, and location of underlying organs and structures. To percuss correctly, place the first joint of your left middle finger on your patient's skin. Keep the rest of your hand poised above the skin, as shown here.

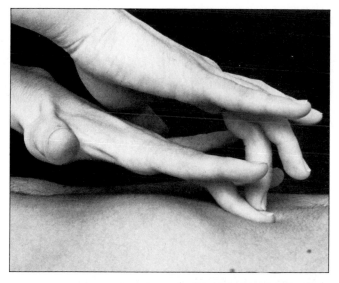

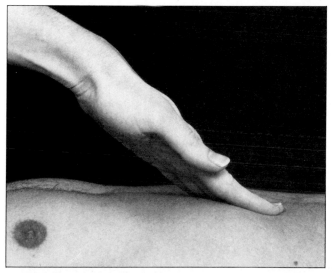

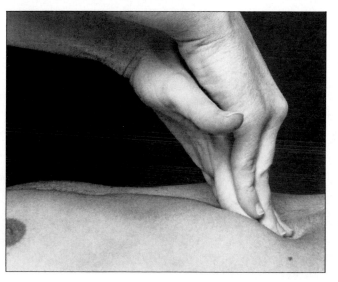

4 Now, tap the left finger with your right middle finger, as shown in this photo. As soon as you've done this, withdraw your right finger so you don't damp the vibration.

Listen carefully as you tap several times. Then, move your hands slightly and repeat the procedure until you've percussed his entire abdomen. Compare the difference in sounds (if any).

Note: If you're left-handed, place your right middle finger on your patient. Tap with your left middle finger.

5 You'll palpate your patient's abdomen to help confirm data that you've gathered from observation. Use light palpation—indenting your patient's skin about ½" (1.3 cm)—to check the skin's temperature and moistness and to detect large tumors and tender or painful areas.

6 Use deep palpation—indenting your patient's skin more than ½"—to locate organs and determine their size, to check for spasticity or rigidity, to feel pulsations, and to detect crepitus and tumors.

☎ *Nursing tip:* To increase your fingertip pressure when palpating, place one hand on top of the other, as shown here.

Remember to record on your patient's chart what you've seen, heard, and felt.

Assessment

How to examine your patient's mouth

1 *Consider this situation: Edward Falcone, a 21-year-old college student complaining of severe abdominal cramps, has been admitted to your unit. You want to assess his GI system. Begin by examining Mr. Falcone's mouth. Here's how:*

First, gather the equipment you'll need: a tongue depressor, penlight, and a glove or finger cot. Then, have your patient sit on a bed or chair. If he's wearing dentures, ask him to remove them.

Explain the examination procedure to Mr. Falcone and reassure him. If your patient's uncooperative, keep your fingers out of his mouth. Instead, use a tongue depressor.

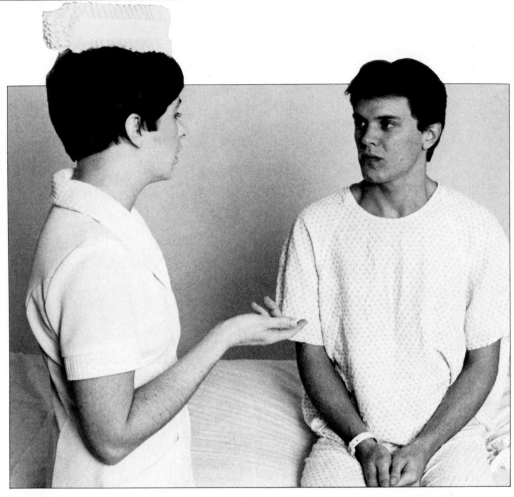

2 Now, observe your patient's lips. They should be pink and smooth. Then, wearing a glove or finger cot, palpate his lips, checking for ulcers, nodules, or lesions. If you notice any, record in your nurses' notes how many, their size and hardness.

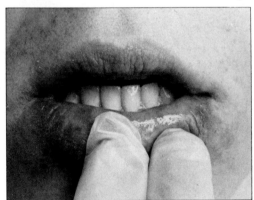

3 Next, instruct Mr. Falcone to open his mouth, so you can examine his gums. To do this, gently push out his right cheek with the tongue depressor. Make sure his gums are pink and moist. If they're not, document in your notes any inflammation, swelling, bleeding, retraction, or distortion.

Then, locate your patient's right parotid duct, which is located inside his cheek, opposite the second molars. Be sure to check the duct for inflammation or drainage.

Now, check the gums and parotid duct on the left side of Mr. Falcone's mouth. Note your observations.

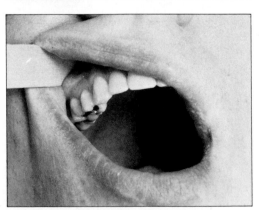

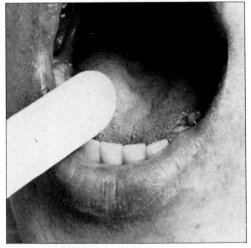

4 Next, inspect his teeth. He should have 32, or 8 on each side of his upper and lower jaws.

With a tongue depressor, tap each tooth on the right side of his mouth. If all's well, Mr. Falcone should feel the tapping in each tooth. Then, tap each tooth on the left side of his mouth.

Remember: If your patient feels pain in any tooth, suspect an abscess. If he doesn't feel anything when you tap, he may have nerve damage.

5 Check for any missing teeth. Note any broken or severely decayed teeth. If your patient has a tooth that looks loose, try to wobble it with your finger or the tongue depressor. If it's extremely loose, recommend he have it extracted as soon as possible.

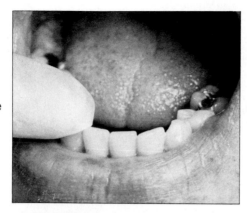

8 Now, have him stick out his tongue. It should appear pink and velvety. Then, carefully inspect the tip and sides of his tongue. If you see any ulcers, growths, or lesions, palpate them to determine their size and hardness.

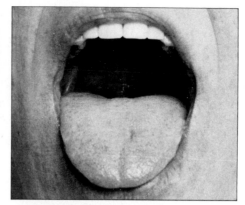

6 Now, check your patient's bite. Have him close his mouth and relax his lips. Open his lips with your fingers. His molars and premolars should touch. His lower canines and incisors should slide slightly inside his upper front teeth.

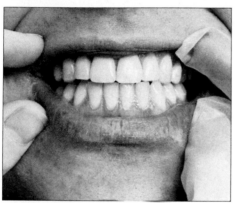

9 Ask your patient to touch the tip of his tongue to the roof of his mouth. Examine the area under his tongue. Make sure the mucous membrane is pink, moist, and smooth. Again, palpate any ulcers, growths, or lesions you see, and note their size and hardness.

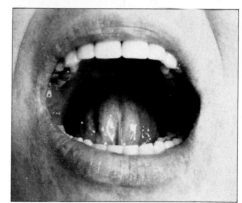

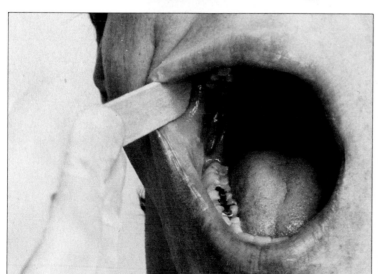

7 Insert a tongue depressor into Mr. Falcone's mouth and hold his right cheek out. With a penlight, examine the upper, lower, and middle buccal membranes inside his right cheek. You'll see smooth, pink pigmentation. Or, if your patient's black, you'll see patchy pink pigmentation.

If you find any ulcers, growths, or lesions, palpate them to determine their size and hardness. Document your findings in your nurses' notes.

Then, examine the membranes on the left side of your patient's mouth.

10 Next, palpate your patient's submaxillary (salivary) ducts, located on either side of the frenulum. They should feel soft and moist. But if you note hardness or irregularities, document your findings.

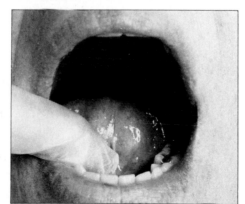

11 Next, hold down Mr. Falcone's tongue with the tongue depressor. Using a penlight, examine the roof of his mouth. The hard palate should be firm and white; the soft palate, pink and cushiony.

Document all observations in your nurses' notes.

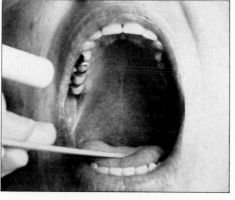

Assessment

How to assess your patient's throat

1 *Let's say you're about to examine Mr. Falcone's throat. Follow these steps:*
First, explain the procedure to your patient. Then, gather the necessary equipment: a tongue depressor, a glove or finger cot, and a laryngeal mirror with an attached light. Now, hold down your patient's tongue with the tongue depressor. Ask him to say "Ah." As he does, locate his uvula, which should be smooth and pink. If his uvula's red and swollen, suspect an allergic reaction.

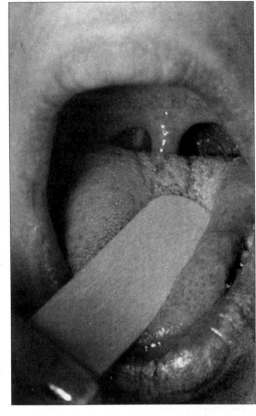

2 Now, locate the fauces, which is the folded tense tissue at the back of his mouth. Look for Mr. Falcone's tonsils on either side of the fauces. The tonsils should look like mottled brown or pink cushions of tissue.
Behind the fauces, you'll observe the pharynx, which should appear pink and smooth in nonsmokers, yellowish-red (with small nodules) in smokers.

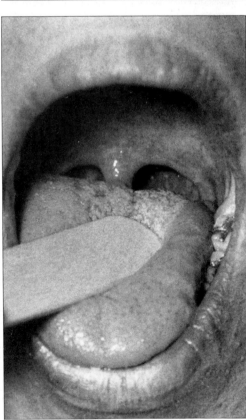

3 Spray a laryngeal mirror with antifog solution, if possible. Next, ask Mr. Falcone to tilt his head back. Insert the laryngeal mirror along the side of his mouth, with the mirror pointing up.
📞 *Nursing tip:* If your patient begins to gag when you place the mirror in his mouth, get a doctor's order for anesthetic throat spray. But, remember, you'll have to stay with your patient until his gag reflex returns.
Shine the light into your patient's posterior nasal cavity. Because the mirror is small, you'll be able to observe only one portion of the cavity at a time, as shown in the illustration.

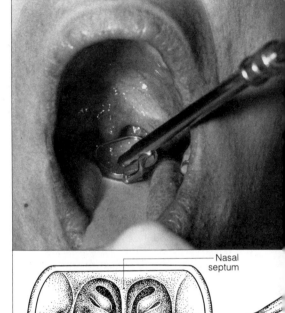

Nasal septum

4 Then, inspect Mr. Falcone's larynx and vocal cords. To do this, angle the laryngeal mirror down your patient's throat. Rest the bent part of the mirror just above his uvula. Locate your patient's pink, moist epiglottis, as shown in the illustration. Note any swelling, ulcerations, or growths in your patient's throat.

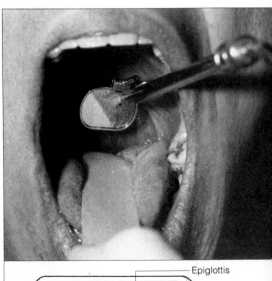

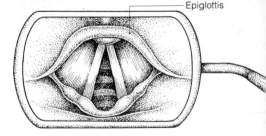

Epiglottis

5 Next, instruct your patient to pronounce an "Ah" or "Eee." As he does, you'll see both his false and true vocal cords. If all's well, his vocal cords will separate as he inhales and come together as he exhales.

Then, carefully look at his vocal cords. They should appear smooth, white, and glistening. If they don't, note any inflammation, discharge, ulcers, or growths.

Finally, document your findings in your nurses' notes.

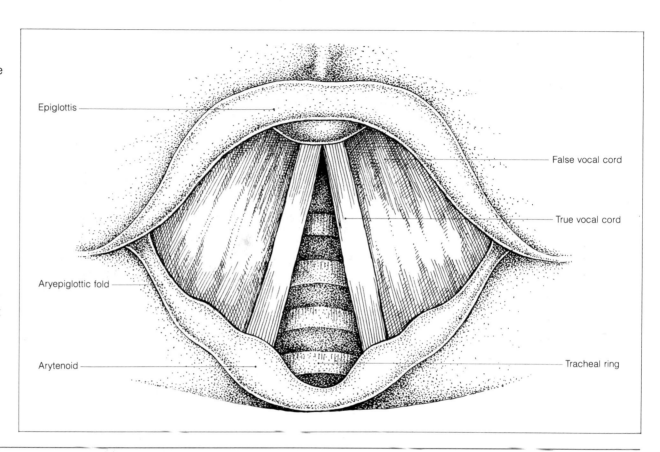

Epiglottis

False vocal cord

True vocal cord

Aryepiglottic fold

Arytenoid

Tracheal ring

How to inspect your patient's abdomen

1 *Preparing to inspect Mr. Falcone's abdomen? If so, follow these guidelines:*

First, ask Mr. Falcone to empty his bladder. Then, thoroughly explain the procedure to him.

Have your patient lie on his back on an exam table in a warm, well-lighted room. To help your patient relax, place one pillow under his head and another under his knees. Instruct him to place his hands at his sides, or on his upper chest, whichever he prefers.

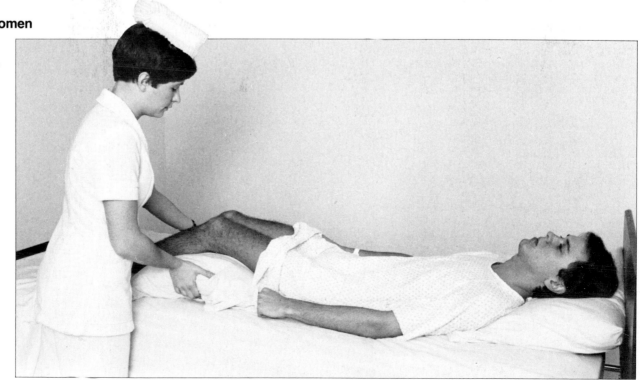

Assessment

How to inspect your patient's abdomen continued

2 Then, expose Mr. Falcone's abdomen from his xiphoid process to his symphysis pubis, as the nurse is doing here. Leave the rest of his body covered, to protect his privacy and keep him warm.

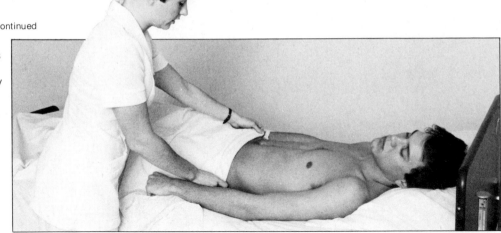

3 Now, check your patient's abdomen for overall symmetry. Is his abdomen flat, round, protuberant, or scaphoid? If his abdomen looks distended, test him for ascites, after you auscultate his abdomen.

Next, examine your patient's skin for unusual pigmentation, rashes, lesions, hair distribution, or dilated veins. Note any striae or abdominal scars from past trauma or surgery. Document in your nurses' notes the appearance and location of any skin abnormalities. (For more information on documenting skin abnormalities, see the *Nursing* PHOTOBOOK *Assessing Your Patients.*)

Also, inspect your patient's abdomen for lumps and masses. Check thoroughly for asymmetry, which may indicate an intra-abdominal mass.

Locate your patient's umbilicus and examine its contour. Is it red or swollen? If you detect a protrusion that yields to moderate fingertip pressure, suspect an umbilical hernia. Also, check for bluish umbilicus (Cullen's sign), which may indicate intra-abdominal hemorrhage.

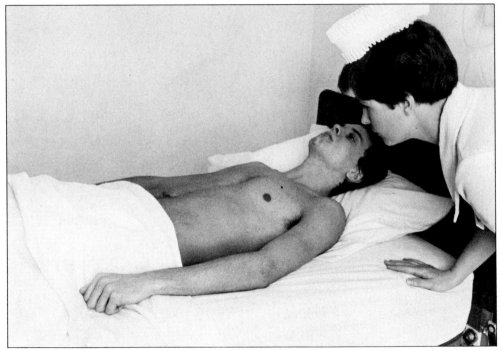

4 Then, examine Mr. Falcone's epigastrium for aortic pulsations. To do this, look across his abdomen at eye level. Note the rate, intensity, and location of the pulsation.

Check your patient's abdomen for peristaltic movement. Normally, you'll see either no motion or a slight wavelike motion across his abdomen. However, if you see undulating waves (especially accompanied by a distended abdomen and cramps), your patient may have an intestinal obstruction.

Be sure to document all of your observations in your patient's records.

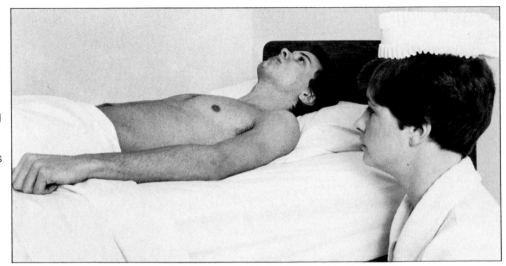

Auscultating your patient's abdomen

1 *Do you know how to auscultate your patient's abdomen? If you're unsure, follow the guidelines below. As you know, you'll auscultate before you palpate, as palpation may change the frequency of your patient's peristaltic sounds.*

First, picture his abdomen divided into quadrants, as shown here.

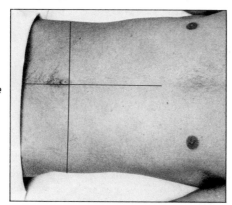

2 Now, explain the procedure to your patient. After warming the stethoscope's diaphragm in your hands, place it on your patient's upper right quadrant, above his umbilicus. You should hear intermittent rumbling and gurgling, which are normal bowel sounds. Count these sounds for 1 minute. If all's well, you'll hear 5 to 34 sounds per minute.

Suppose you hear loud bowel sounds occurring more frequently than 34 per minute. Your patient may have a hyperperistaltic, non-obstructed bowel.

If you hear frequent, high-pitched, tinkling bowel sounds, or gurgling rushes and loud splashes, your patient may have a bowel obstruction.

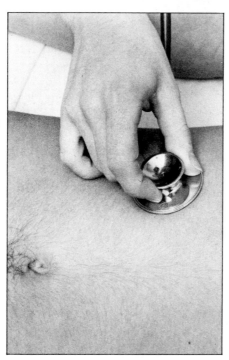

3 What if you don't hear any bowel sounds? Then, auscultate each quadrant, in clockwise order, for 2 to 5 minutes—or until you hear something. If you still don't hear anything in any of the quadrants, your patient may have a paralytic ileus.

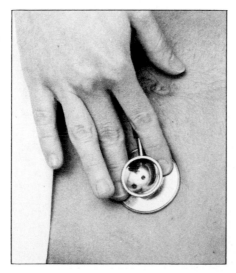

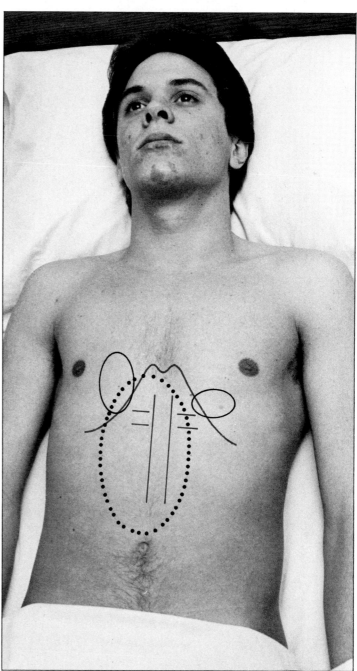

4 Now, use this photo as a guide to auscultate for friction rubs, bruits, or venous hums. Auscultate by moving the stethoscope at 2″ to 3″ (5 to 7.6 cm) intervals in each area.

Friction rubs sound like two pieces of leather rubbing together. If you hear friction rubs over your patient's liver and spleen, suspect a hepatic tumor or splenic infarct.

As you know, bruits have a purring sound. If you hear bruits in your patient's abdomen, suspect an aortic aneurysm or partial arterial obstruction.

A continuous medium-pitched sound indicates a venous hum. If you hear a venous hum in your patient's abdomen, he may have hepatic cirrhosis.

Assessment

How to percuss and palpate your patient's abdomen

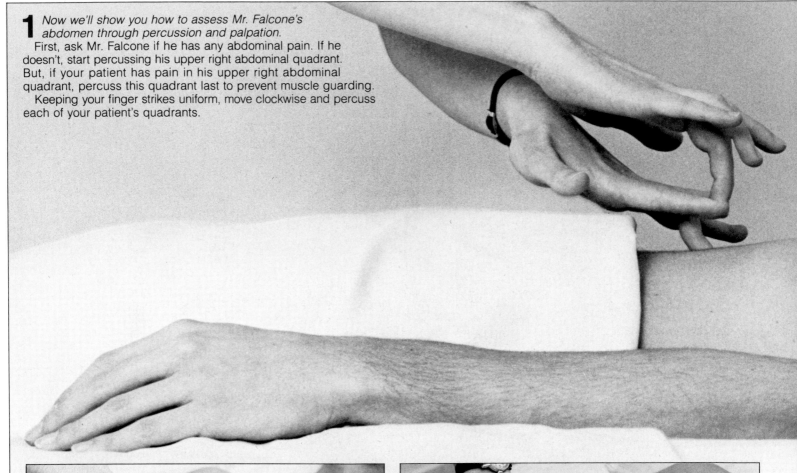

1 *Now we'll show you how to assess Mr. Falcone's abdomen through percussion and palpation.*
    First, ask Mr. Falcone if he has any abdominal pain. If he doesn't, start percussing his upper right abdominal quadrant. But, if your patient has pain in his upper right abdominal quadrant, percuss this quadrant last to prevent muscle guarding.
    Keeping your finger strikes uniform, move clockwise and percuss each of your patient's quadrants.

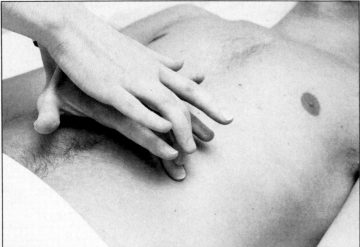
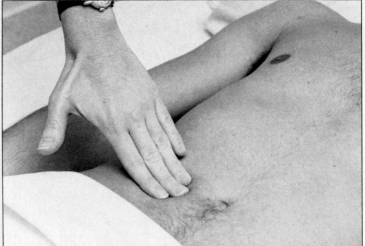

2 As you percuss each abdominal quadrant, mentally note where the percussion sounds change from tympanic to dull. This helps you identify the location of abdominal organs and detect possible masses.
    Remember, a dull sound in your patient's suprapubic area may indicate a distended bladder.

3 Now, *lightly* palpate Mr. Falcone's abdomen, following the same clockwise order used for percussion. Note his skin temperature. In addition, check for tenderness and possible masses.
    (For more information on light and deep palpation, see the *Nursing* PHOTOBOOK *Assessing Your Patients*.)

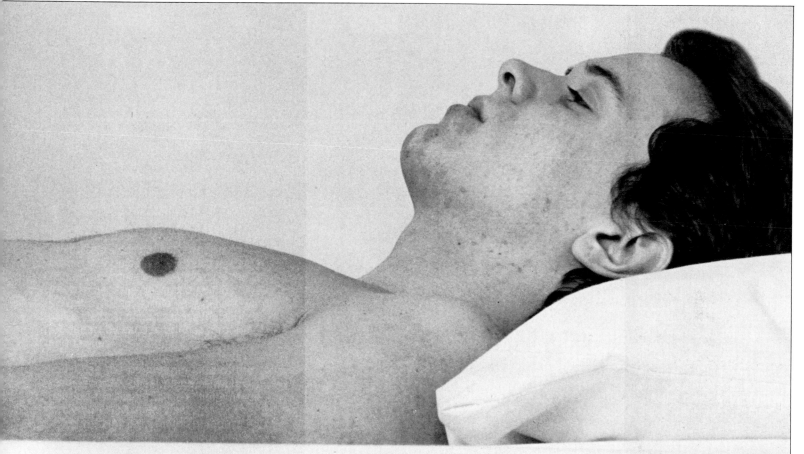

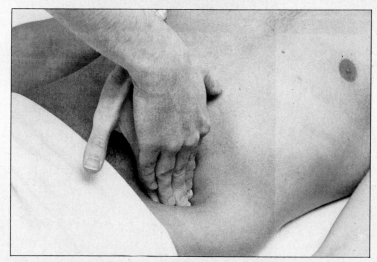

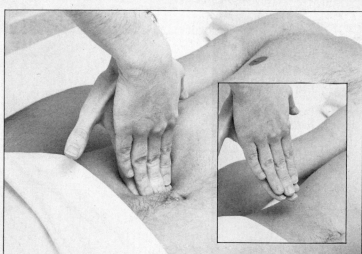

4 Next, *deeply* palpate Mr. Falcone's abdomen, following the same clockwise order. Check for organ enlargement, masses, bulgings, or swellings. If you detect a mass in your patient's abdomen, note its location, size, shape, consistency, tenderness, and mobility. Then, document any pulsations you may feel.

5 If you detect a tender or painful area in your patient's abdomen, check for rebound tenderness, which may indicate peritoneal inflammation. To do this, slowly push your fingertips into the tender area.
[Inset] Then, quickly release them. If your patient feels a sharp pain when you release your fingers, he has rebound tenderness. Finally, document all observations in your nurses' notes.

Assessment

How to assess your patient's liver

1 *In this photostory, we'll show you how to properly assess Mr. Falcone's liver. Before you begin, explain the procedure to your patient.*

Starting near his umbilicus, percuss upward, following his right midclavicular line. Stop when you hear the percussion sounds change from tympanic to dull. The dull sound means you've located the lower border of your patient's liver. Mark this point with a felt-tip pen or a stick-on dot, as the nurse is doing here.

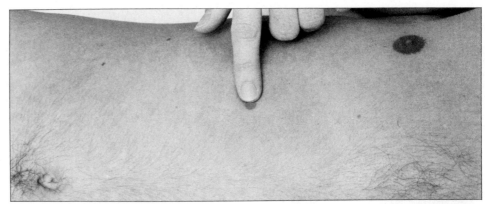

2 Now, place your fingers over the patient's right midclavicular line at midsternal level. Percuss downward, following his midclavicular line. Stop when you hear the percussion sounds change from resonant to dull. The dull sound means you've located the upper border of his liver. Mark this point, as before.

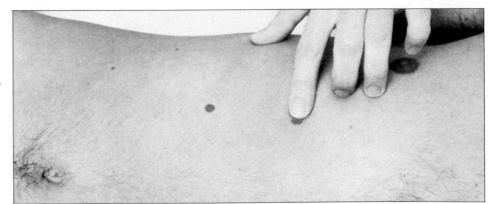

3 Then, measure the distance between the two points. The distance should range anywhere from 2⅜" (6 cm) to 4¾" (12 cm). If your patient's liver measures more than 4¾" (12 cm), or seems large for his body build, he may have an enlarged liver.

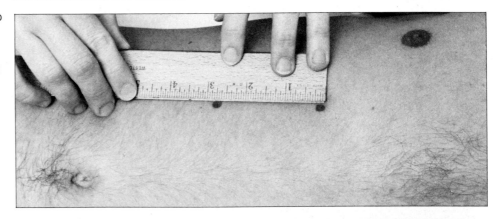

4 If you suspect an enlarged liver, repeat the percussion procedure at your patient's midline. The distance between the upper and lower liver borders should be 1¾" to 3¼" (4.4 cm to 8.3 cm).

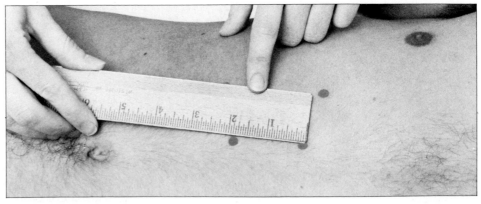

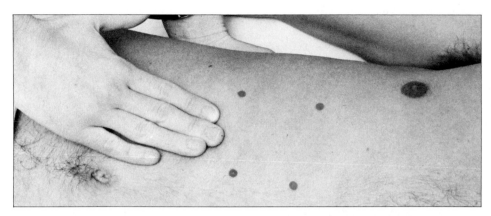

5 Now, deeply palpate the lower edge of Mr. Falcone's liver, using the bimanual technique. To do this, stand at his right side. Place your palm under his back, directly under his 11th and 12th ribs. Then, place your right hand on his abdomen, parallel to his midline. Your right hand should be below the stick-on dots marking his liver's lower border.

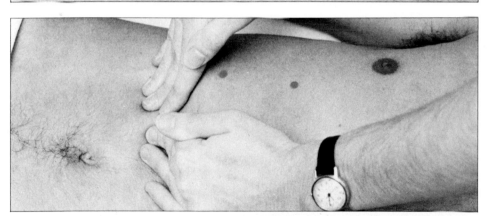

6 Ask your patient to breathe deeply through his mouth. As he exhales, press downward with your right fingers and upward with your left. Each time he exhales, try to push a little deeper, until you feel the liver's lower edge. If all's well, you'll feel a sharp, firm, regular ridge.

But, in some cases, you may feel only an increased resistance against your fingertips, indicating the liver's lower edge. If you've reached the maximum palpation depth and still can't feel your patient's liver, move your right hand closer to the right costal margin. Repeat the palpation procedure, until you feel the liver's lower edge, meet increased resistance, or conclude that the liver's not palpable.

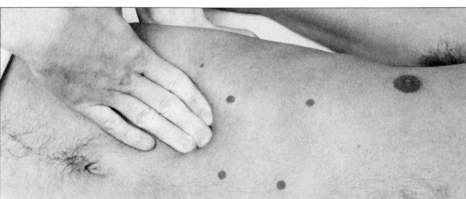

7 Or, you may prefer to use the hooking technique to palpate Mr. Falcone's liver. To do this, stand at your patient's right side, facing his feet.

Place the fingertips of both your hands on his abdomen, just below the dots marking his liver's lower border.

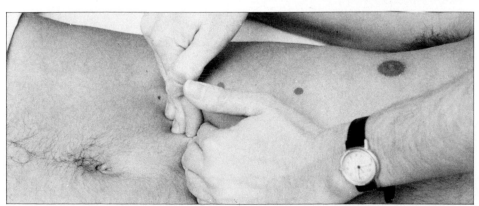

8 Then, push down, and carefully draw your fingers toward the right costal margin. Ask your patient to breathe deeply. As he exhales, you may feel the liver's lower edge or increased resistance.

Finally, document your findings in your nurses' notes.

Assessment

How to assess your patient's stomach and spleen

1 *Are you assessing Mr. Falcone's stomach and spleen? If so, follow this procedure:*

First, thoroughly explain the procedure to your patient and re-assure him that you'll be gentle. Make sure the room's warm and well lighted. Your patient should be lying on his back on the exam table with his hands at his sides (or on his upper chest).

Now, percuss slightly above and to the right of Mr. Falcone's umbilicus. Continue to percuss across his abdomen to his left anterior axillary line. Note the area where the sound changes from dull to tympanic. As you know, a tympanic sound means you're percussing over his stomach.

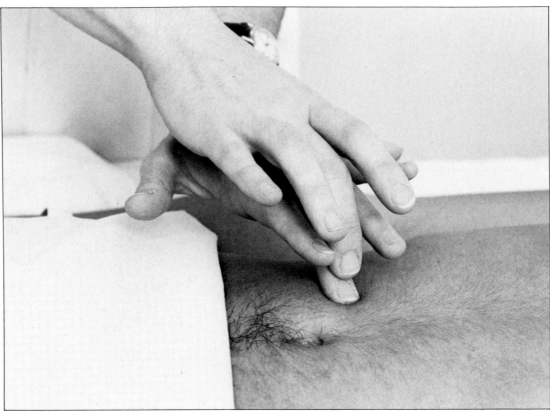

2 Then, move your fingers slightly above and to the right of your patient's umbilicus. Percuss across his abdomen, about 2″ (5 cm) above the area where you first percussed. Again, note where the percussion sound changes from dull to tympanic, and compare these findings to the first percussion line.

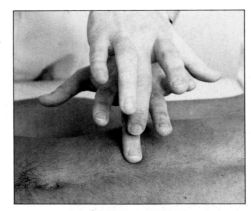

3 Now, continue this procedure until you've percussed Mr. Falcone's entire stomach and determined its approximate size and position. *Remember:* The size of your patient's stomach may vary greatly within the normal range.

If more than five sixths of your patient's stomach is left of the median line, and his upper abdomen is distended, suspect an abnormally enlarged stomach. These findings may indicate a tumor or intestinal obstruction.

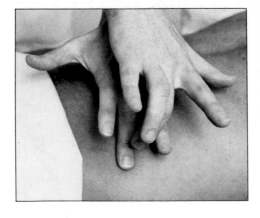

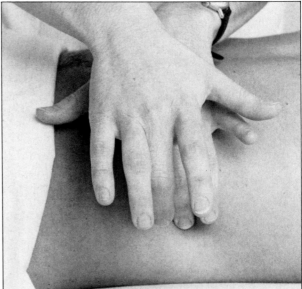

4 Next, you'll percuss your patient's spleen. To do this, move your fingers to the area just under your patient's left midaxillary line. Starting above the 12th rib (at the 11th intercostal space), percuss each interspace up to the 8th rib (the 7th intercostal space). If your patient's spleen is normal, you'll hear a tympanic sound as you percuss. If his spleen's enlarged, you'll hear a dull sound.

5 Suppose you don't detect splenic enlargement. Then, locate and percuss your patient's 9th intercostal space at the left anterior axillary line. As you percuss, you should hear tympany.

Now, instruct your patient to take a deep breath as you percuss the same area. If you hear the percussion sound change from tympanic to dull as he inhales, suspect an enlarged spleen.

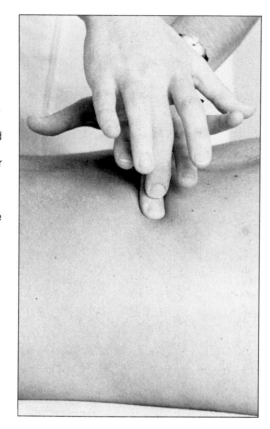

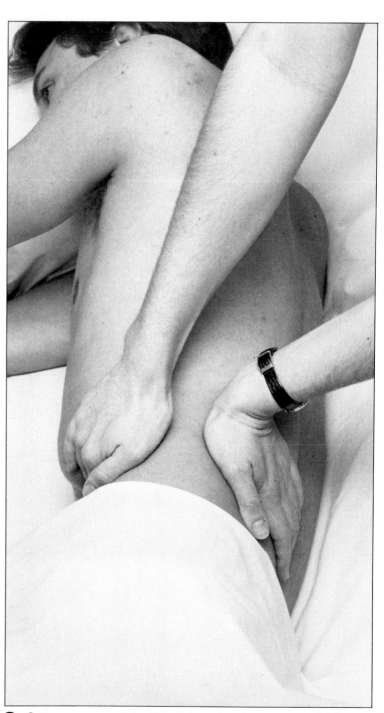

6 Here's how to palpate Mr. Falcone's spleen. Place your left hand under his lower left rib cage. Then, gently press your right fingers against his lower left costal margin.

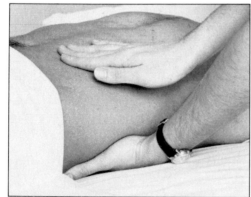

7 Now, instruct your patient to breathe deeply. As he does, push up with your left hand and press down with your right fingers. If you feel the spleen's edge, the spleen is probably enlarged about three times its normal size. Note the spleen's shape and consistency.

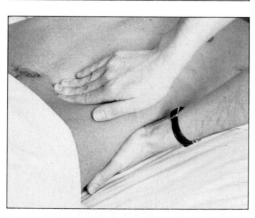

8 Suppose you can't feel Mr. Falcone's spleen when he's lying on his back. Have him turn onto his right side and flex his knees and hips forward. Repeat the palpation, following the same procedure.

Finally, if you detect any splenic enlargement, document it as slight, moderate, or great. As you know, slight enlargement is enlargement of ½″ to 1¾″ (1.3 to 4.4 cm) below the costal margin. Enlargement of 1¾″ to 3¼″ (4.4 to 8.3 cm) is classified as moderate. Enlargement of 3¼″ (8.3 cm) or more is considered great.

Document all findings in your nurses' notes.

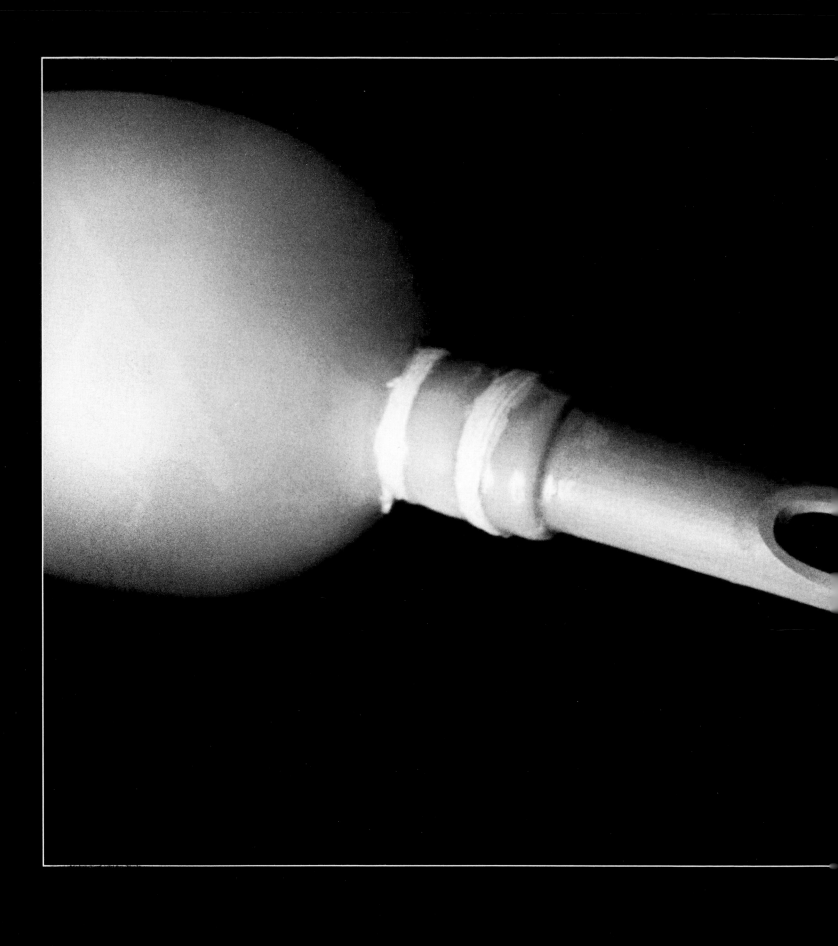

Managing Esophagogastric Disorders

Special problems

Nasogastric tube care

Gastrostomy care

Special problems

What's the first thing you think of when someone says esophagogastric disorder? Do you think of a patient with GI bleeding or esophageal varices? Do you know when the doctor may order a cervical pharyngostomy or a Sengstaken-Blakemore tube? Do you know how to assist in these insertion procedures? Or how to care for a patient with these tubes in place?

What if the doctor orders total parenteral nutrition (TPN) for your patient? Do you know how to administer it? Can you name five TPN additives? Do you know how to change the TPN tubing properly?

As you can see, there's more to caring for a patient with an esophagogastric disorder than you may have thought. Read the next few pages. In them, you'll not only find the answers to these questions, but you'll find important instructions and helpful tips for dealing confidently with these special problems.

Nurses' guide to esophagogastric disorders

Has it been a while since you've cared for a patient with an esophageal or gastric disorder?

Remember, with any esophagogastric disorder, you must explain all procedures to your patient and reassure him and his family as much as possible. Obtain a complete medical history. Also, remember to teach your patient proper medication and dietary management, if applicable. Read the chart carefully.

Disorder	Signs and symptoms	Possible causes	Nursing considerations
Achalasia (failure of gastro-esophageal sphincter to relax)	• Vomiting • Dysphagia • Ache or burning pain in lower esophagus • Dilated esophagus and impairment of gastroesophageal sphincter.	• Cause unknown, but most common in patients between ages 20 and 40	• Instruct patient to chew his food thoroughly. • Keep patient in high Fowler's position after eating. • Tell patient to avoid eating for 2 to 3 hours before bedtime. • Elevate head of patient's bed 6″ (15 cm). • Be prepared to assist doctor with esophageal dilation. Or, prepare your patient for surgical myotomy to loosen gastroesophageal sphincter.
Mallory-Weiss syndrome (massive hemorrhage from laceration of gastroesophageal junction)	• Sudden, acute, massive hematemesis • Nausea • Hypotension • Low hematocrit	• Prolonged or forceful vomiting • Associated with chronic alcoholism	• Closely monitor patient's postural vital signs. • Begin I.V. therapy (normal saline solution, plasma, blood), as ordered. • Be ready to perform iced gastric lavage, as ordered. • Draw blood for hemoglobin and hematocrit levels, as ordered. • Be prepared to assist with upper GI endoscopy, as ordered. • If hemorrhage is not self-limiting, be ready to prepare patient for surgery, as ordered.
Reflux esophagitis	• Heartburn • Regurgitation of gastric contents • Painful or difficult swallowing • Chest tightness or pain • Hematemesis or melena	• Hiatal hernia • Weak gastroesophageal sphincter pressure • Prolonged nasogastric intubation • Increased intra-abdominal pressure • Surgical resection of gastroesophageal junction, or myotomy	• Administer medications, as ordered. • Tell patient to avoid the following: wearing tight clothing, eating before bedtime, reclining after meals, and bending over. • Elevate head of patient's bed 6″ (15 cm). • Urge patient not to smoke, if applicable. • Give patient small, frequent feedings that are high in protein and low in fat. Avoid foods that stimulate gastric acid secretions, such as alcohol, caffeine, and fatty foods. • Instruct patient to chew food thoroughly.
Peptic ulcer disease (PUD)	• Gnawing or burning epigastric pain an hour after meals • Pain relieved by food or antacid. • Pain wakens patient at night. • Feeling of fullness • Hematemesis or melena	• Stress (contributing factor) • Hypersecretion of gastric acid (determined through gastric analysis) combined with a decrease in mucosal protective factors, such as mucus production • History of prolonged use of aspirin, alcohol, corticosteroids, or caffeine	• Administer medications, as ordered. • Frequently give patient antacids and small amounts of food to help relieve GI distress. • Encourage patient not to smoke, if applicable. • Provide diet that eliminates substances known to increase acid secretion, such as caffeine, alcohol, and fatty foods. • Be alert for signs and symptoms of gastric perforation: sudden, intense, epigastric pain; possible referred pain to one or both shoulders; tender abdomen with muscle guarding; and diminished or absent bowel sounds.
Gastric carcinoma	• Vomiting • Feeling of fullness; weight loss; anorexia • Constipation; diarrhea • Indigestion • Anemia • Hematemesis or melena • Weakness; fatigue; epigastric discomfort	• Cause unknown, but may be hereditary or dietary	• Prepare patient for subtotal or total gastrectomy, as ordered. • Watch for postsurgical signs of wound complications, such as purulent, foul-smelling drainage, inflammation, or dehiscence, and signs of pulmonary complications (shortness of breath and increased pulmonary secretions). • Encourage turning, deep breathing and coughing, to prevent pulmonary complications. • Administer pain medication, as ordered. • Treatment for inoperable cases aimed at symptom relief.

Nurses' role in upper GI endoscopy

Whenever the doctor suspects an esophageal or gastric inflammation, ulceration, or tumor, he'll order upper GI endoscopy for your patient. As you probably know, upper GI endoscopy provides visualization of the esophageal and gastric mucosa, and the upper duodenum. It's also used to obtain specimens for lab analysis.

To prepare your patient for this procedure:
• restrict his food and fluid intake for at least 6 hours prior to the test, or as ordered.
• explain the examination to him. Emphasize the importance of each step, as it's done. Be prepared to administer sedatives, such as diazepam (Valium*), or meperidine (Demerol*), as ordered.
• remove his dentures, if applicable.
• spray his throat with a local anesthetic, such as Cetacaine (as ordered) to minimize gagging. Or, if he can, have him gargle with the anesthetic.
• place him in a side-lying position and put a small pillow under his head to make him more comfortable.

Important: Have suction and emergency cardiopulmonary resuscitation (CPR) equipment on hand in case your patient develops respiratory or cardiac problems during the examination.

As the examination progresses, monitor your patient's vital signs. Also, label any specimens and send them to the lab for analysis.

When the examination's completed, make your patient as comfortable as possible. Also, remember these important points:
• Monitor your patient for 24 hours. Stay alert for bleeding, dysphagia, fever, and neck, chest, or abdominal pain, any of which may indicate esophageal, gastric, or duodenal perforation. Notify the doctor immediately if there are complications.
• Have your patient stay in a side-lying position (or place him in this position) and restrict his food and fluid intake for about 2 hours, or until his gag reflex returns. To test for gag reflex return, touch the back of his throat with a cotton-tipped applicator or tongue blade; use a short, quick motion. If no response occurs, wait about 30 minutes and test again.
• After his gag reflex returns, encourage your patient to suck on hard candy or throat lozenges to reduce throat irritation. After 2 to 4 hours, he'll be ready to resume his normal diet. Document everything in your nurses' notes.

Sengstaken-Blakemore tube insertion: Your role

1 *Forty-year-old Tanya Natske was admitted to the ICU 3 hours ago with bleeding esophageal varices. At that time, the doctor ordered vasopressin (Pitressin*) administered at a rate of 0.2 units per minute. Because the vasopressin failed to adequately control the hemorrhage, the doctor's ordered a Sengstaken-Blakemore tube. She'll expect you to assist with the insertion.*

Begin by explaining the insertion procedure to Ms. Natske, and reassure her. Then, ask a coworker to closely monitor your patient's vital signs as you gather this equipment: Rusch Sengstaken-Blakemore (S-B) tube, nasogastric (NG) tube, irrigation set, water, piston syringe, emesis basin with ice, large basin, pressure manometer (mercury sphygmomanometer), water-soluble lubricant, penlight, four hemostats, small sponge block or football helmet, Hoffman clamp, and adhesive tape.

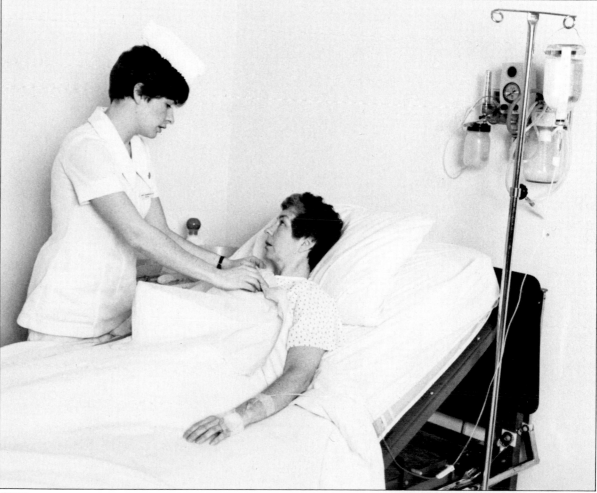

*Available in both the United States and in Canada

Special problems

Sengstaken-Blakemore tube insertion: Your role continued

2 Now, test the S-B tube's gastric and esophageal balloons for leaks by inflating each of them with a syringe. Then, submerge the balloons in a basin of water. Stay alert for any escaping air bubbles.

Run water through the S-B and NG tubes to check tube patency.

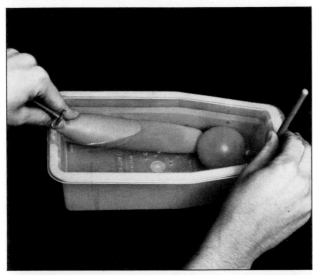

3 Lay the S-B and NG tubes side by side so the tip of the NG tube's positioned just above the S-B tube's esophageal balloon.

Use the NG tube to measure the distance from the S-B tube's esophageal balloon to the S-B suction lumen. With tape, mark the correct length on the NG tube. You'll use the NG tube to aspirate oral secretions and to check for bleeding above the esophageal balloon, as ordered.

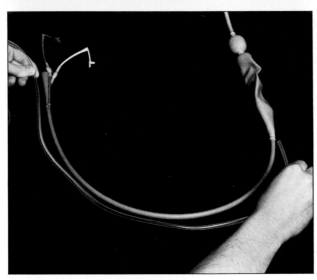

4 Place Ms. Natske in a semi-Fowler's position, with her neck hyperextended.

Note: If your patient's unconscious, place her in a left side-lying position. Elevate the head of the bed at least 15°.

As ordered, chill the S-B and NG tubes in a basin of ice, which stiffens them, making insertion easier. Administer sedatives, as ordered.

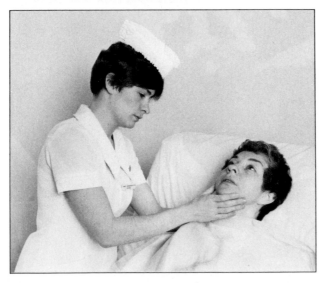

5 Use a penlight to inspect Ms. Natske for any nasal deformities. To do this, alternately press each of her nostrils shut, and ask her to inhale through her open nostril. Tell the doctor which nostril seems more patent. If your patient has a nasal obstruction, the doctor may insert the S-B tube orally.

Apply water-soluble lubricant to the S-B and NG tubes.

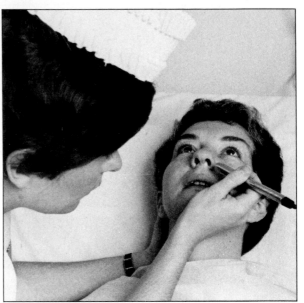

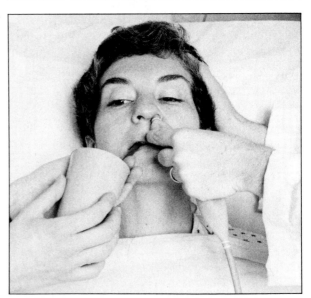

6 The doctor will twist both balloons around the S-B tube and begin insertion. As she inserts the tube, encourage your patient to breathe through her mouth.

When the doctor advances the first balloon into the patient's nostril, tell your patient to begin swallowing. To prevent gagging, have her sip water through a straw, chew ice, or dry swallow. Continue to reassure her.

7 When the S-B tube's entered Ms. Natske's stomach, aspirate her gastric contents with a bulb syringe, as the nurse is doing here. Document the amount, color, and consistency of return.

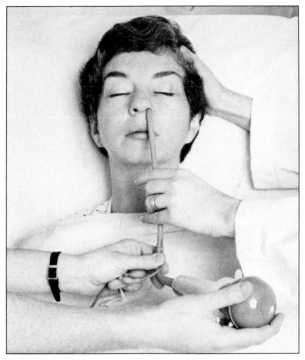

8 Now, you'll insert an NG tube into the other nostril and advance it toward the lower esophagus (see pages 46 to 51 for insertion guidelines). Continue inserting the tube until you reach the tube's premeasured mark, which indicates the tube's in your patient's lower esophagus.

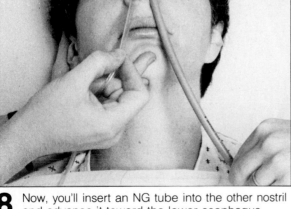

9 Once in place, tape the NG tube to Ms. Natske's cheek.

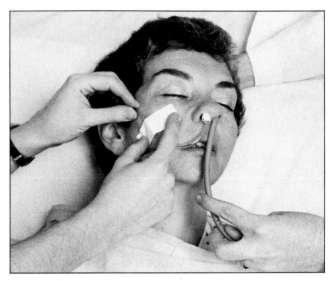

10 Before proceeding, the doctor may order portable X-rays of the lower chest and upper abdomen to confirm tube and balloon placement.
If everything's okay, you're ready to inflate the S-B tube's gastric balloon (in some hospitals, this is the doctor's responsibility). Use a piston syringe to infuse 250 to 500 cc of air into the balloon, as ordered.

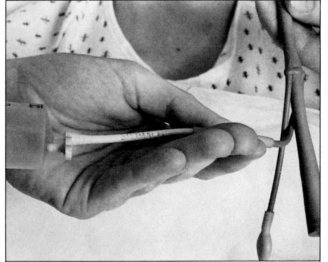

11 Using hemostats, double clamp the gastric balloon's intake port.

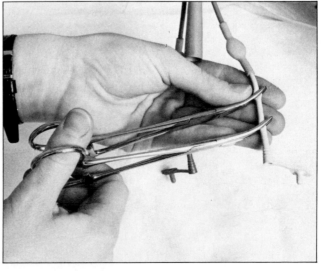

Special problems

Sengstaken-Blakemore tube insertion: Your role continued

12 Apply gentle traction to the S-B tube by positioning a small sponge block around the tube, under you patient's nose. Then tape the S-B tube to the sponge.

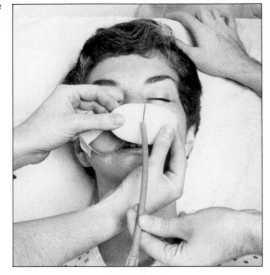

13 Alternately, slide a football helmet over your patient's head. Tape the S-B tube to the helmet's mouth guard.

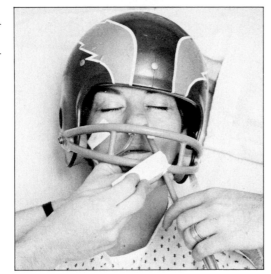

14 To inflate the esophageal balloon, insert a Y-connector into the correct lumen opening. Attach the mercury manometer to one side of the Y-connector.

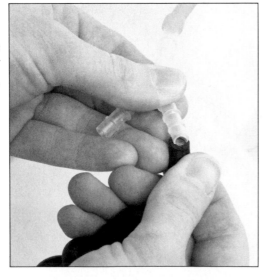

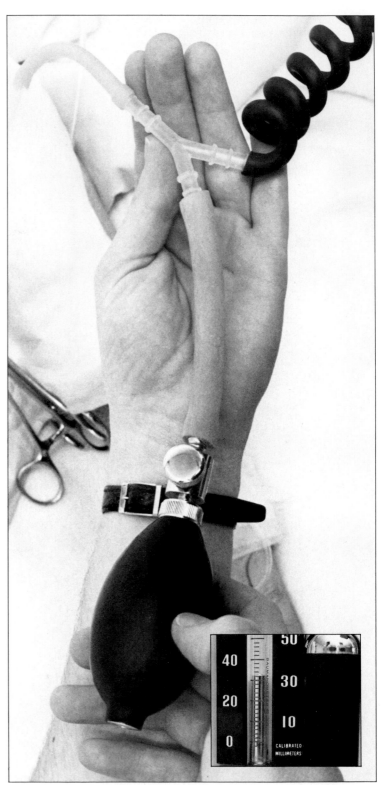

15 Attach the manometer's inflation bulb to the Y-connector's other side.
Inflate the balloon with 30 to 40 mm Hg air pressure, as ordered (see inset).

16 Double clamp the tubing. Label the lumen with the amount of inflation pressure used.

Closely monitor your patient and the tube's lumen pressure. *Remember:* Never leave a patient with an S-B tube unattended.

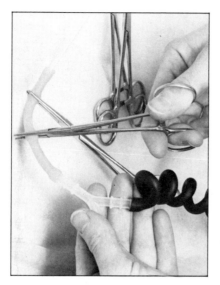

17 *Important:* Tape a pair of scissors to the head of your patient's bed. If she develops signs of acute respiratory distress while the S-B tube's in place, pinch the tube at your patient's nose. Then, cut the tube approximately 3" (7.5 cm) from this point, to deflate the balloons. Withdraw the tube, and notify the doctor.

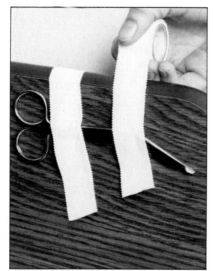

18 Connect intermittent gastric suction to the large suction lumen. Irrigate this lumen hourly, or as ordered.

Or, lavage your patient's stomach with 500 ml of normal saline solution, through the suction lumen.

Record the amount, color, and consistency of the aspirated material.

In addition, be prepared to administer a neomycin sulfate (Mycifradin Sulfate*) or saline-solution enema, as ordered, to help prevent your patient from developing ammonia intoxication.

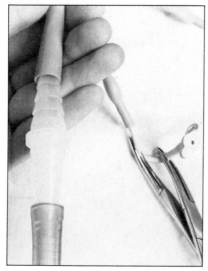

19 As ordered, draw venous blood to determine electrolyte balance, CBC, type and crossmatch. And as shown in this photo, draw arterial blood to determine blood gas measurements. Prepare to give whole blood transfusions, if needed.

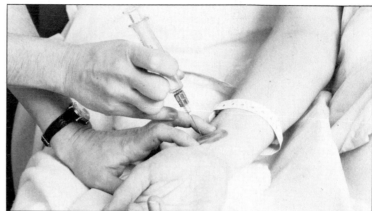

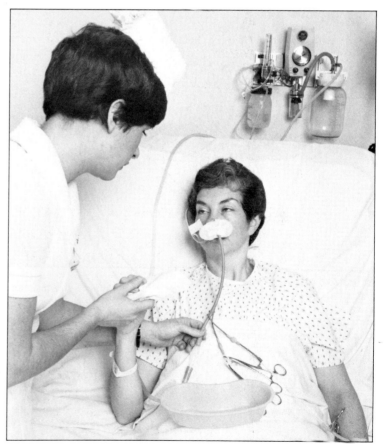

20 Keep your patient as warm and comfortable as possible. Clean Ms. Natske's nostrils frequently. Apply water-soluble lubricant to each nostril.

In case of oral secretions, place a basin on your patient's lap and have some tissues handy.

If after several hours the bleeding's still uncontrolled, prepare your patient for surgery, as ordered.

Document everything in your nurses' notes.

*Available in both the United States and in Canada

Special problems

How to care for a patient with a cervical pharyngostomy

Under most circumstances requiring a nasogastric (NG) tube, you'll pass the tube through one of your patient's nostrils, as ordered by the doctor. Once inserted, the tube may be used alternately for feedings and gastrointestinal suction. But, if you're caring for a patient who'll need an NG tube for a long period of time, the doctor may perform a cervical pharyngostomy.

If this is the case, the doctor will make a small incision over your patient's pyriform sinus. He'll use this incision to create a tube tract from the pyriform sinus to the esophagus. Then, the doctor will pass a well-lubricated NG tube through the incision, into your patient's stomach. After the tube's inserted, he'll check the tube's position, suture the tube to the patient's skin, and apply a sterile dressing.

What's your role in cervical pharyngostomy? First, gather the necessary equipment. Then, explain the procedure to your patient in words she can understand. Try to make her as comfortable as possible. Assist the doctor, as ordered.

When the tube's inserted, remember to:
• check the tube's position before each feeding (see page 52 for details).
• check the suture site frequently for redness or discharge. If you see either, notify the doctor.
• change the dressing at least every 24 hours, or immediately if soiled. Clean the area around the tube, using a solution that's half hydrogen peroxide and half sterile water. Then apply povidone-iodine ointment, using aseptic technique.
• give good mouth care.
Between feedings, keep the tube clamped. Cover the end of the tube with a sterile gauze pad. Wrap a rubber band around the pad. Then, loop the tube on top of the dressing. To prevent the tubing from being pulled out, tape it to the dressing, as shown here. Document everything in your notes.

Nursing tip: Encourage your patient to suck on some hard candy to reduce throat irritation.

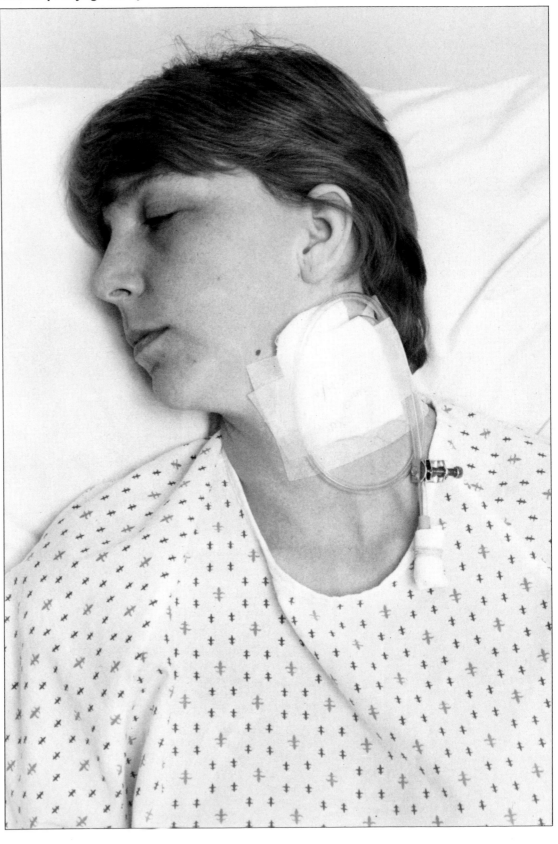

Understanding total parenteral nutrition (TPN)

Total parenteral nutrition (TPN), frequently referred to as hyperalimentation, is an intravenous infusion of nutrients given to a patient who can't get adequate nutrition through his GI system. But, TPN is contraindicated for a patient who:
• is terminally ill and has had all therapy discontinued.
• suffers from hypercoagulation or bleeding abnormalities.
• has an obstructed or partially thrombosed superior vena cava.

Naturally, your patient will accept TPN more readily if you explain the reason behind it. Try to anticipate and answer his questions. Tell him how the solution's prepared, how it's administered, and how much it will limit his activities.

TPN ingredients

TPN is a mixture of 50% dextrose in water, amino acids, and special additives (see the chart below). The mixture must be prepared under a laminar flow hood in your hospital's pharmacy.

Most TPN solutions have similar amounts of amino acids and 50% dextrose in water. However, the solution's additives may vary according to your patient's needs.

After the correct solution has been delivered to your unit, refrigerate it until the therapy begins.

Important: Before administering TPN solution, always check its expiration date. In most cases, TPN solution must be used within 24 hours of preparation.

How TPN is administered

TPN enters your patient's bloodstream through one of three insertion sites: direct central line, central line through peripheral vein, or central line through jugular vein.

Usually, you'll administer TPN through a large, deep vein, as ordered by the doctor. Doing so dilutes the solution with a greater blood flow. *Note:* Use a pump to keep the infusion rate constant.

As you probably know, your patient's body will need time to adjust to TPN because it's a highly osmolar solution. So, following doctor's orders, administer 10% dextrose in water before you begin administering TPN. Then, after the adjustment period, begin administering TPN at a *slow* rate. Gradually increase the infusion rate (as ordered) until the desired rate is achieved.

Remember, always monitor your patient closely when he's receiving this therapy. (For guidelines, see page 40.)

(For guidelines, see page 40.)

Learning about TPN components

Wondering how the doctor decides which additives to include in your patient's total parenteral nutrition (TPN) solution? First, he'll determine your patient's metabolic needs by assessing his physical condition and performing blood studies. Then, he'll prescribe a combination of additives in varying amounts, which will help your patient meet these needs.

To help you understand the specific function of TPN additives, study this chart.

TPN additive	Purpose
50% dextrose in water	Provides calories needed for metabolism
Amino acids	Supply protein needed for tissue repair
Potassium	Necessary for cellular activity and tissue synthesis
Folic acid	Essential for DNA formation
Vitamin D	Necessary for maintenance of serum calcium levels and for bone metabolism
Vitamin B complex	Aids in final absorption of carbohydrates and protein
Vitamin K	Needed to help prevent bleeding disorders
Vitamin C	Necessary for wound healing
Sodium	Helps control water distribution to maintain fluid balance
Chloride	Used to regulate the acid-base equilibrium and maintain osmotic pressure
Calcium	Promotes blood clotting and aids teeth and bone development
Phosphate	Minimizes the threat of peripheral paresthesia
Magnesium	Helps absorb carbohydrates and protein
Acetate	Needed to prevent metabolic acidosis
Trace elements (zinc, cobalt, manganese)	Necessary in wound healing and red blood cell synthesis

Using protein-sparing solutions

If your patient's nutritional needs require fewer amino acids than those commonly found in total parenteral nutrition (TPN) solution, the doctor may administer a protein-sparing solution. This solution contains the same amount of vitamins, electrolytes, and minerals as TPN, but only half the amount of amino acids. And, instead of the 50% dextrose found in a normal TPN solution, the protein-sparing solution contains 10% dextrose or less. The reduced amount of dextrose and amino acids in the solution permits irritation-free infusion through the patient's peripheral vein. Sometimes the doctor will supplement this solution with an I.V. fat emulsion to provide additional calories for the patient. (For information on I.V. fat emulsion, see the *Nursing* PHOTOBOOK *Managing I.V. Therapy.*)

The doctor may order a protein-sparing solution for a patient who's had major surgery or acute trauma, or for the patient who's receiving chemotherapy or radiotherapy. Don't administer protein-sparing solution to patients suffering from shock, or cardiac, renal or hepatic failure.

When caring for a patient receiving protein-sparing solution, observe these guidelines:
• Always use aseptic technique when changing the dressing or I.V. setup.
• Maintain an even flow rate.
• Check the insertion site frequently for tenderness, redness, or edema, any of which may indicate phlebitis (chemical and septic), or extravasation. Remove the catheter and insert a new one at another site. Be sure to document your observations and notify the doctor.

Important: As you know, if extravasation goes unchecked, it may result in tissue sloughing or necrosis.

Special problems

Caring for a patient receiving total parenteral nutrition (TPN)

To properly care for a patient receiving TPN, you'll need to provide emotional as well as physical support. Reassure your patient and his family throughout the therapy, and answer all of their questions. In addition, follow these guidelines:

• Monitor your patient's vital signs at least once every 4 hours.

• Weigh your patient at the same time each day to check his fluid balance. Always use the same scale and make sure he's wearing the same clothing.

• Document your patient's daily caloric intake. Keep accurate intake and output records.

• Draw blood to determine electrolyte balance, osmolarity, blood sugar, creatinine, and blood urea nitrogen (BUN) levels.

• Provide good mouth care. Instruct your patient to brush his teeth and gargle several times a day.

• Most important, test your patient's urine sugar, acetone, and specific gravity every 6 hours.

To determine his urine sugar and acetone levels, perform a dipstick test. If test results show a urine sugar level of 2+ or greater—or if you discover a high acetone concentration—notify the doctor. In these situations, the doctor may increase the TPN solution's insulin level, or order sliding-scale insulin coverage administered subcutaneously.

If, following testing, the specific gravity of your patient's urine is not the normal level (1.020), the doctor may change the infusion rate or the TPN solution's contents.

During TPN therapy: Caring for the patient with a central I.V. line

Caring for a patient receiving total parenteral nutrition (TPN) therapy through a central I.V. line? In such a case, your patient's weakened condition and the TPN solution's high sugar content make him more susceptible to infections; for example, *Candida* (fungal), *Staphylococcus aureus* or *S. epidermidis*, or *Klebsiella*. You can reduce his chance of developing one of these infections, and other complications, by following these guidelines:

• Always follow strict aseptic technique when caring for your patient's central I.V. line, or when changing his dressing.

• Change the entire I.V. setup every 24 to 48 hours (depending on your hospital's policy). But, if the catheter begins to leak or any part of the equipment becomes contaminated, change the setup immediately.

• Change the dressing at least three times a week.

• Never use the TPN line to do a central venous pressure (CVP) reading, piggyback any solution, or take a blood sample.

• Closely monitor the infusion rate to avoid metabolic complications such as hyperglycemia or electrolyte imbalance. Use an infusion pump to keep the rate constant. Never infuse the solution too rapidly or attempt to catch up if the infusion is behind schedule. Doing so may cause a fluid overload.

• Check your patient for signs and symptoms of thrombophlebitis: pain or soreness in his neck, shoulder, or chest; neck vein distention; or swelling of his catheterized arm. If any of these occur, notify the doctor.

• Notify the doctor if your patient shows signs of infection: redness, swelling, oozing pus at the catheter site, or a sudden temperature rise.

Suppose your patient develops an infection. If your hospital policy allows, remove the catheter, using strict aseptic technique. Remember to cut off 1″ to 2″ (2.5 to 5 cm) of the catheter tip with sterile scissors. Then, put the catheter tip in a sterile test tube or container, and send it to the lab for analysis. (For more information on removing a TPN catheter, see the *Nursing* PHOTOBOOK *Managing I.V. Therapy.*)

How to change TPN tubing

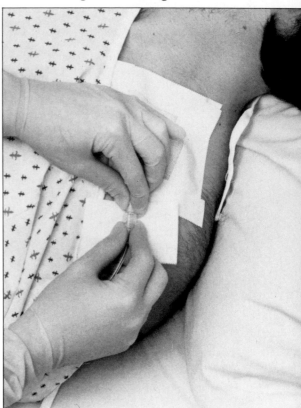

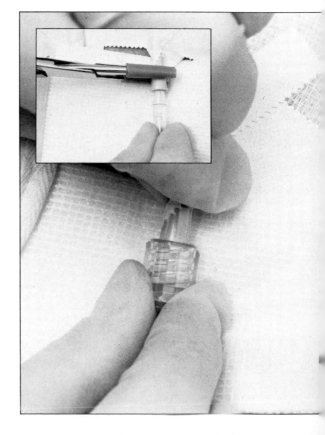

1 *Let's say your patient's re-ceiving total parenteral nutrition (TPN) therapy. As you know, you must change his tubing every 24 to 48 hours, according to your hospital's policy. Here's how:*

Begin by explaining the procedure to your patient. Place him flat on his back. Make sure the prepared TPN solution, including clean, primed tubing, is hanging within reach.

Then, wash your hands thoroughly. Put on a pair of sterile gloves.

Now, place a 2"x2" sterile gauze pad under the catheter connection, creating a sterile field, as shown here.

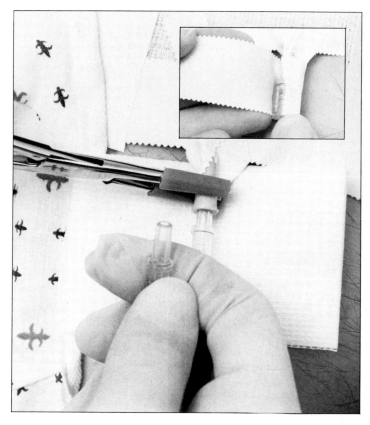

3 Next, rotate the tubing until it detaches from the hub. Quickly insert the new primed tubing into the hub, as shown here. Screw the Luer connection onto the catheter's hub.

[Inset] Tape the connection, making sure it's secure.

2 Before you disconnect the tubing, unscrew the Luer connection (if you're using one).

[Inset] Then, keeping the hub catheter steady with a hemostat, disconnect the tubing.

Now, ask your patient to perform Valsalva's maneuver. Doing so will create internal pressure and make an air embolism less likely. But remember, a Valsalva maneuver is contraindicated for a patient with a cardiac disorder.

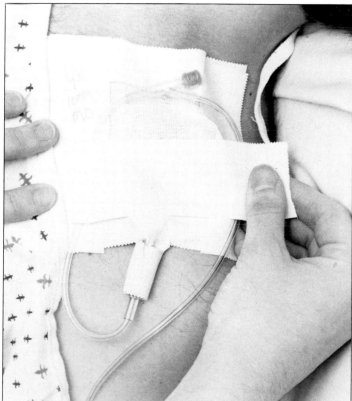

4 To prevent the tubing from being dislodged accidentally, loop the tubing on top of the dressing and tape it, as shown here. Discard the old bottle and tubing. Encourage your patient to relax as much as possible during therapy.

Finally, document the procedure in your nurses' notes.

Special problems

For the patient receiving TPN: How to change the dressing

1 *Whenever you care for a patient receiving total parenteral nutrition (TPN), you must change her dressing at least three times a week. But, if the dressing becomes wet or loose, change it immediately. Here's how:*

First, gather the necessary equipment: disposal bag for soiled dressing, 4"x4" gauze pads, face masks for you and your patient (according to your hospital's policy), povidone-iodine applicator and ointment, acetone, sterile gloves, and nonallergenic tape.

Place a face mask over your patient's mouth, if she must wear one. Then, slip on your mask.

Caution: Never put a face mask on a patient who needs oxygen or who has a nasogastric tube in place.

Now, using proper handwashing technique, wash and dry your hands. Remember, you'll maintain aseptic technique throughout the procedure.

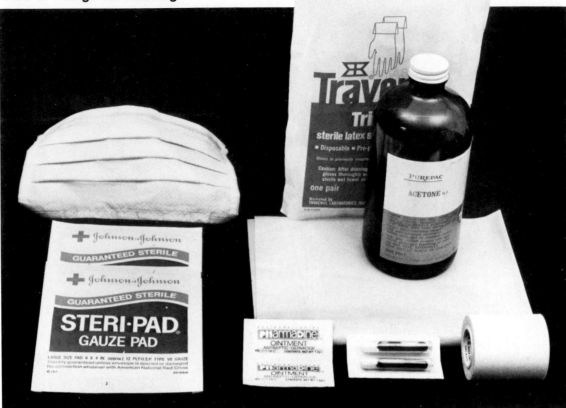

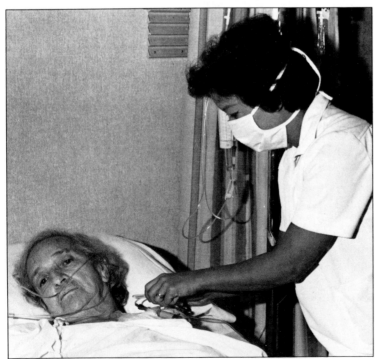

2 Now, explain the procedure to your patient and place her in a supine position. For better access to the insertion site, turn her head to one side. Doing so also reduces the risk of contamination from the patient's oropharynx.

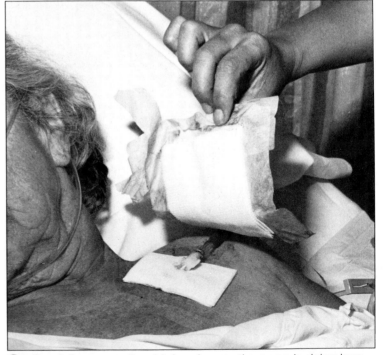

3 Carefully remove the old dressing, as the nurse is doing here. As you do this, pinch together the dressing's soiled surfaces so they don't contaminate your hands.

Place the soiled dressing in the disposal bag.

4 Next, examine the insertion site for signs of infection, such as discharge, inflammation, or soreness. If any drainage is present, obtain a specimen for culture and label it with your patient's name, her hospital identification number, the date, and the time. Send the specimen to the lab and notify the doctor.

Make sure the catheter's positioned correctly. If the catheter's taped in place, remove the soiled tape.

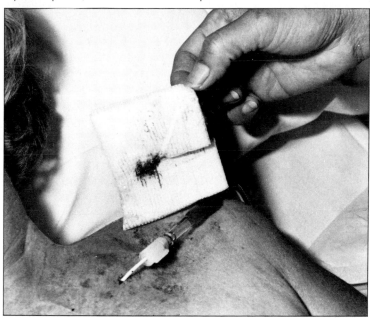

6 Next, clean the site with the povidone-iodine applicator, using the same circular motion. Allow the povidone-iodine to dry naturally. Don't fan the site with your hands. Doing so increases the risk of contamination.

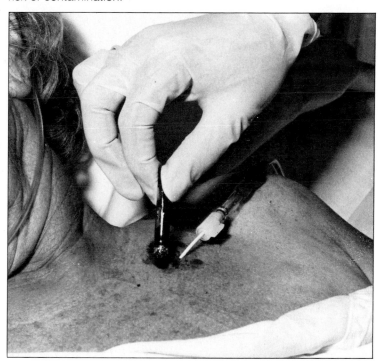

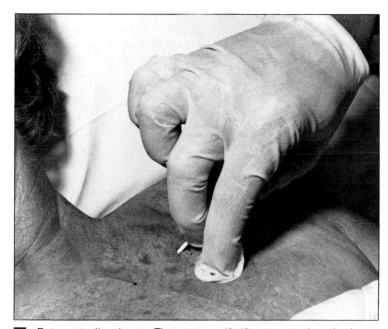

5 Put on sterile gloves. Then, use a 4"x4" gauze pad soaked with acetone to clean the area around the insertion site. Use a circular motion, working from the site outward.

As you work, take care not to touch the catheter with the acetone. Doing so could corrode it.

If the acetone does contact the catheter, wipe the catheter immediately with sterile saline solution.

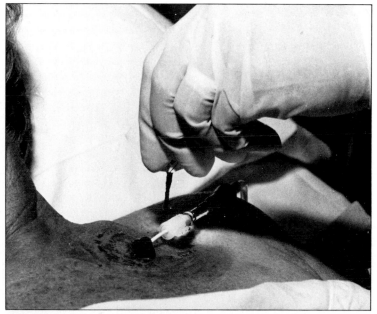

7 Now, apply povidone-iodine ointment to the insertion site. If the catheter isn't sutured, tape it in place, using the chevron taping method. (For complete details on taping a TPN catheter, see the *Nursing* PHOTOBOOK *Managing I.V. Therapy.*)

Remove the soiled dressings from your patient's room. Discard them, according to your hospital's policy. Document the procedure in your notes.

Nasogastric tube care

Do you know how to insert a nasogastric (NG) tube properly? How to check NG tube placement? How to care for a patient with an NG tube in place? How to irrigate an NG tube? If not, you'll need to read the information on these pages.

We've also included information on various types of tubes, as well as brands of tube feeding solutions for those of you who'll use NG tubes to administer feedings.

You also discover how to use a nasogastric tube to perform gastric lavage (regular and iced); and learn how to obtain specimens for gastric analysis.

Nurses' guide to nasogastric (NG) tubes

Do you know when and how to use each of the following NG tubes? The chart which follows gives you specific instructions, and outlines your nursing responsibilities. Study it carefully.

In addition, remember these general guidelines when caring for a patient with any type of NG tube:
• Before inserting the tube, use running water to check the tube's patency.
• Provide good mouth care.
• Keep patient's nostrils well lubricated.
• Use proper taping techniques to prevent irritation of skin and nasal passages.
• Stay alert for signs of tube-feeding intolerance: nausea, vomiting, and diarrhea. If you observe any, stop feeding and notify the doctor. You may be administering the feeding too rapidly.

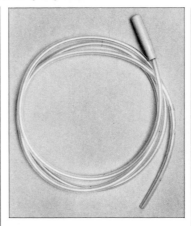

Bard-Parker™ stomach tube (Levin-type)

Description
• A 50″ (127 cm) long, clear plastic tube with holes at tip and along side

Use
• Aspiration of gastric contents
• Administration of tube feedings

Nursing actions
• If tube's too limp to insert easily, chill it in a basin of ice. If tube's too stiff, make it more pliant by heating it in a basin of warm water.
• To keep tube patent, irrigate it once every 2 hours with 30 ml of normal saline solution.
• Attach tube to intermittent low suction or use straight bag drainage, as ordered.
• Before beginning tube feeding, verify tube placement, using the tests described on page 52.
• Start half-strength tube feedings at a rate of 25 ml an hour, or as ordered. Increase to full-strength solution within 24 hours.

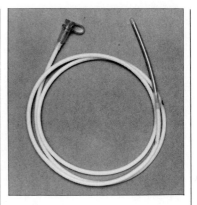

Nutriflex™ nasogastric feeding tube

Description
• A 30″ (76 cm) long, radiopaque Erythrothane® polyurethane tube with mercury-weighted tip to aid in insertion
• Distal portion treated with Hydromer™ dry coating, which, when moistened, provides lubrication for easier insertion.

Use
• Administration of tube feeding

Nursing actions
• Use feeding tube placement stylet to stiffen tube for easier insertion.
• Before inserting stylet, inject about 10 ml water into tube to activate inner feeding-tube lubricant.
• Before insertion, moisten end of tube to activate lubricant.
• Confirm tube placement before initiating tube feeding. (Use guidelines on page 52.)
• If tube feeding won't be continuous, irrigate the tube with 20 ml water in a 50 cc syringe to remove possible blockages. Do this before administering feeding solution.
• Never use a syringe smaller than 50 cc to irrigate the tube. Excessive pressure from a small syringe may cause tube to rupture.
• Never use an infusion pump that delivers pressures greater than 40 pounds per square inch (psi). Bursting strength of feeding tube is 80 psi.
• For initial feeding, administer water for 2 to 4 hours or until you note patient's tolerance to tube and infusion.
• Start half-strength tube feedings at a rate of 25 ml hour, or as ordered. Increase to full-strength solution within 24 hours.
• After the tube's removed, dispose of the mercury-weighted tip, according to your hospital's policy.

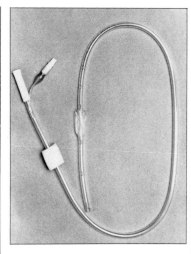

G. Moss™ nasoesophageal gastric decompression tube

Description
• Double-lumen, 35″ (90 cm) long, clear plastic tube with X-ray (radiopaque) tip and foam rubber cushion at nasal opening

Use
• Aspiration of gastric contents

Nursing actions
• Before inserting, make sure balloon's intact.
• Insert tube completely and verify its placement in patient's stomach before inflating the balloon.
• Inflate balloon with 30 cc air.
• Withdraw excess length of catheter from nostril, positioning balloon at the cardia. Then, secure sponge against nostril to prevent tension.
• Apply intermittent or continuous suction, as ordered.
• To ensure tube patency, irrigate tube with 30 ml normal saline solution every 2 hours.

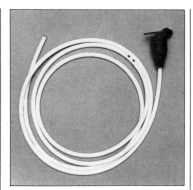

Keofeed® silicone-rubber feeding tube

Description
• A 42″ (107 cm) long, soft silicone-rubber tube weighted at distal end with a short column of mercury.
• Available in small French sizes to provide patient comfort for long-term tube feedings. Tube marked at 25, 50, and 75 centimeters from distal end.

Use
• Administration of tube feeding
• May be advanced to duodenum for intestinal feeding.

Nursing actions
• Use Keofeed monofilament guide to stiffen tube for easier insertion.
• Before inserting guide, inject water-soluble lubricant into feeding tube.
• Check tube placement before initiating tube feeding, as described on page 52.
• For initial feeding, administer water for 2 to 4 hours, or until you note patient's tolerance to tube and infusion.
• Start half-strength tube feeding at a rate of 25 ml per hour, or as ordered. Increase to full-strength solution within 24 hours.
• After the tube's removed, dispose of the mercury-weighted tip, according to your hospital's policy.

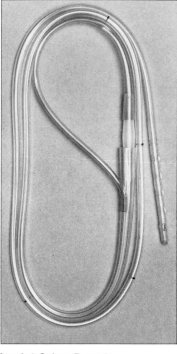

Argyle® Salem Sump®

Description
• Double-lumen, 48″ (122 cm) long, clear plastic gastric tube with a blue sump port and markings at 18, 22, 26, and 30″
• Radiopaque Sentinel Line® for X-ray confirmation of placement
• Gastric suctioning occurs along sides and tip of tube.

Use
• Aspiration of gastric contents
• Administration of tube feedings
• Sump port helps keep stomach mucosa from being drawn into tube during suctioning.

Nursing actions
• Instill only air into sump port.
• Connect clear port to straight bag drainage, intermittent or continuous suction, or clamp it, as ordered.
• Keep tube patent by instilling 30 ml of normal saline solution through clear port every 2 hours.
• Inject air through blue sump port after each irrigation.
• For initial feeding, administer water for 2 to 4 hours, or until you note patient's tolerance to tube and infusion.
• Start half-strength tube feedings at a rate of 25 ml an hour, or as ordered. Increase solution to full strength within 24 hours.

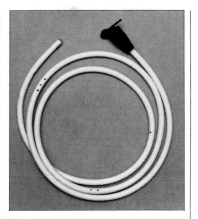

Hedeco Silsoft™ gastrointestinal suction tube

Description
• Single-lumen, 42″ (107 cm) long, radiopaque, silicone-rubber tube with gelatin tip for ease of insertion
• Available in size 16 French with markings at 25, 50, and 75 centimeters.

Use
• Aspiration of gastric contents
• Administration of tube feeding

Nursing actions
• Insert Keofeed tube guide to help stiffen tube and make insertion easier.
• Attach lumen to intermittent low suction, or use straight bag drainage, as ordered.
• Before tube feeding, verify correct tube placement, using tests described on page 52.
• Follow same insertion procedure used for NG tube (see pages 46 to 51).
• For initial feeding, administer water for 2 to 4 hours or until you note patient's tolerance to tube and infusion.
• Start half-strength tube feedings at a rate of 25 ml per hour, or as ordered. Increase to full-strength solution within 24 hours.

Nasogastric tube care

How to insert a nasogastric (NG) tube

1 *Keith Einhorn, a 33-year-old meat cutter suffering from a bowel obstruction, arrives in your unit. The doctor orders the insertion of a nasogastric (NG) tube. If your hospital allows, do you know how to insert one?*

Before you begin, wash your hands thoroughly to help prevent contamination. Then, gather this equipment: size 12 to 18 French NG tube or a Salem Sump® tube, penlight, Hoffman clamp, cup of water with a straw, bulb syringe, piston syringe (optional), paper towel, water-soluble lubricant, gauze pads, nonallergenic tape, bed-saver pad, tincture of benzoin, emesis basin, stethoscope, tissues, normal saline solution, a small rubber band, and a safety pin.

Note: If your patient's an infant, he'll need a small nasogastric tube, size 6 to 8 French. For an older child, use a larger tube, size 8 to 12 French.

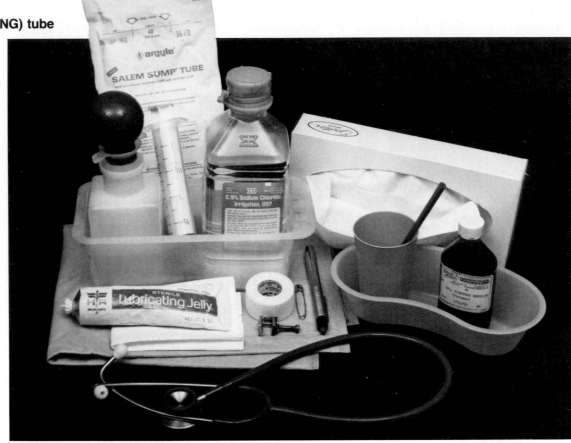

2 Now, test the tube's patency by running water through it. Check it for rough spots and ragged edges.

Using a vinyl plastic nasogastric tube? You may find it too stiff to insert gently. If so, place it in warm water for several minutes to increase its flexibility.

Suppose the tube seems too pliant. Chill it in a basin of ice.

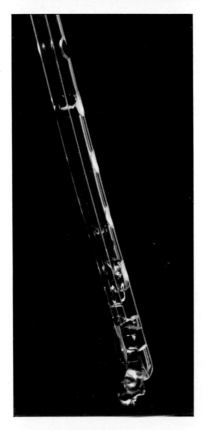

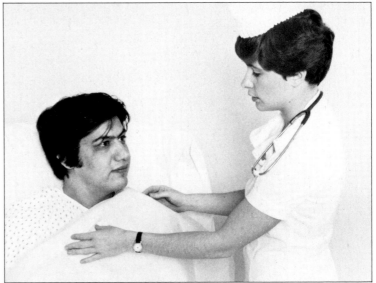

3 Now, explain the procedure to your patient and reassure him. Encourage him to ask questions and answer them completely. Tell him that he may feel some discomfort during the procedure, and agree on a signal he can use to stop it momentarily. This will give him a sense of control.

Next, place your patient in a sitting or high Fowler's position. Cover his gown and the bed linen with bed-saver pads to protect them from spills. Hand him several tissues, as the procedure may stimulate tearing. Also, give him the emesis basin to hold.

4 Using a penlight, examine his nostrils for possible obstructions or deformities. Ask the patient if he has a deviated septum or ever had a broken nose. Then, alternately press each of his nostrils closed and instruct him to inhale through the open nostril. If both nostrils are mechanically obstructed, stop immediately and notify the doctor. He may want you to pass the tube orally. Otherwise, begin the procedure.

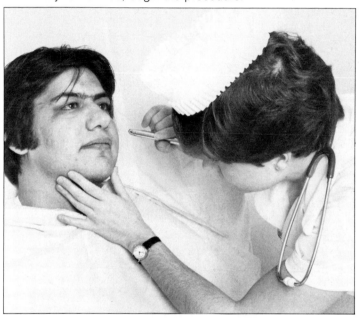

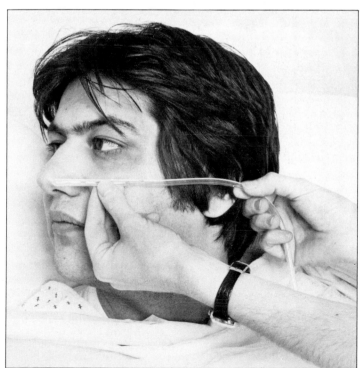

5 Now, follow this two-step method to determine how much tube to insert. First, use the tube to measure the distance from your patient's earlobe to the tip of his nose, as shown here.

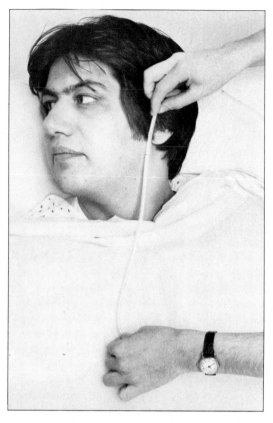

6 Then, measure the distance from his earlobe to the base of his xiphoid process. Total these measurements, and use adhesive tape to mark this length on the tube. Suppose your patient's a child. You'll measure the distance from his earlobe to the tip of his nose. Then, measure from his earlobe to a point midway between his xiphoid process and his umbilicus. Add these measurements and mark the tube, as described.

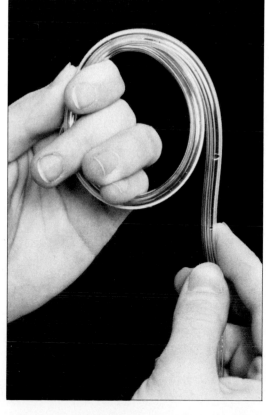

7 To determine the tube's natural curve, hold it about 6" (15.2 cm) from its tip and roll it between your fingers. If no curve is evident, shape a curve yourself by tightly coiling the first 5" (12.7 cm) of tubing around your fingers, as the nurse is doing here.

Nasogastric tube care

How to insert a nasogastric (NG) tube continued

8 Lubricate the first 6" (15.2 cm) of the tube with water-soluble lubricant.

Caution: Never lubricate an NG tube with mineral oil or petroleum jelly. Your patient may aspirate it and develop respiratory complications.

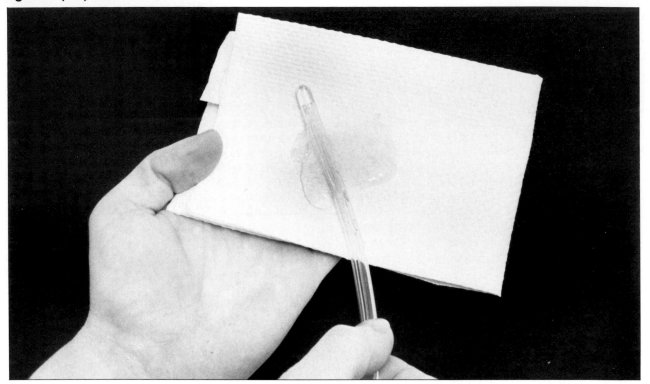

9 Now, have your patient hold his head still as you insert the NG tube into an unobstructed nostril. Gently advance it along the nasal passage toward the posterior nasopharynx. To make this easier, direct the tube toward your patient's ear on that side, not toward his other nostril.

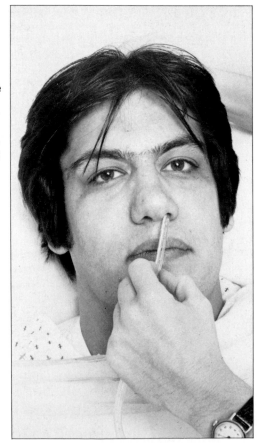

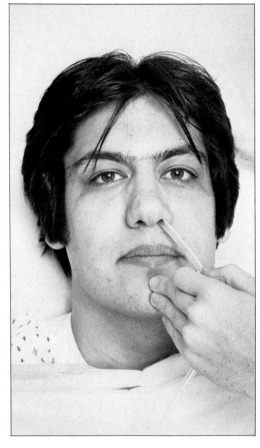

10 When you feel the tube approaching your patient's nasopharynx, rotate it 180° inward, toward his other nostril. Then, continue to advance the tube gently, until it's in the nasopharynx, pointing toward the esophagus.

Important: If you meet resistance at any point, immediately stop advancing the tube. Then, rotate the tube between your fingers about 180°. Try advancing it again. If you're still unable to advance the tube, withdraw it completely. Then, relubricate the tube and try inserting it in the other nostril, provided it's unobstructed.

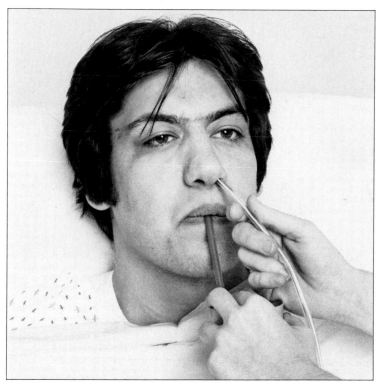

11 What if your patient starts to gag as the tube enters his nasopharynx? Stop advancing the tube immediately and tell your patient to take several deep breaths. Or, if he's allowed to drink water, ask him to take a few sips of water through a straw. Either method will relax his pharynx and calm his gag reflex. Water will also help lubricate the tube.

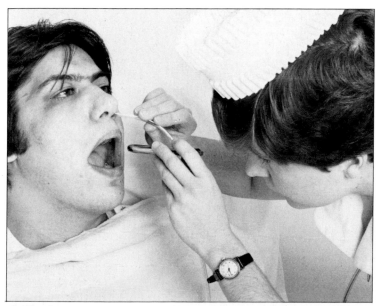

12 Suppose your patient continues gagging. Check his mouth with the penlight to see if the tube is coiled in his mouth or throat. If it is, withdraw the tube until it's straight. Then, let your patient rest for a few moments before continuing the procedure.

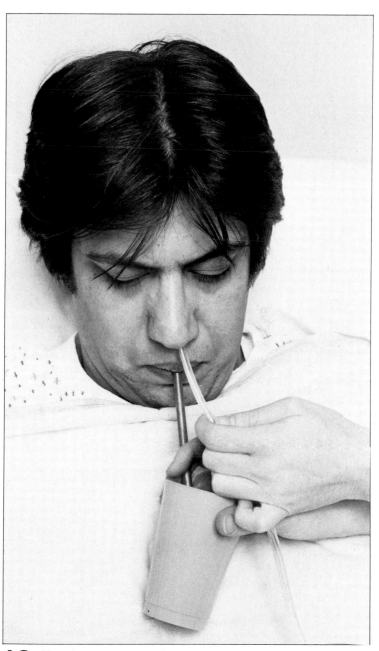

13 Now, instruct your patient to move his head forward so his chin touches his chest. This helps to close his trachea and open his esophagus. Tell your patient to swallow, and continue to advance the tube into his esophagus.

Ask him to sip water as you advance the tube into his stomach. Or, have him chew ice chips. Advance the tubing 3″ to 5″ (7.6 to 12.7 cm) each time he swallows.

Note: If he can't drink water, instruct him to dry-swallow at your signal. *Never give liquids to an unconscious patient.*

Continue inserting the tube until you've reached the premeasured mark. If the tube won't advance that far, you may have inserted it into your patient's trachea, not his esophagus. Or, the tube may have curled in the back of his throat. Withdraw the tubing until it's straight, and try again to insert it correctly.

Nasogastric tube care

How to insert a nasogastric (NG) tube continued

14 At this point in the procedure, you'll want to make sure the tube's in your patient's stomach, not his bronchus. To do this, try at least two tests to check for proper tube placement (see page 52).

When you're sure the tube's properly positioned in his stomach, cut a 3″ (7.6 cm) strip of 1″ (2.5 cm) wide nonallergenic tape. Split the tape lengthwise, leaving a small tab intact at one end.

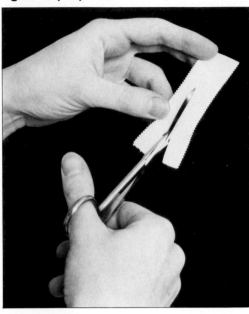

16 Now, connect the sump port to the suction port, using a connector like the one shown here.

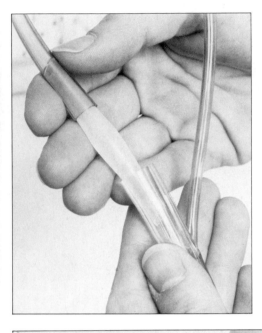

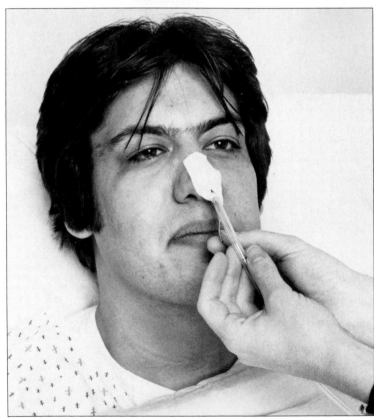

15 Now, apply tincture of benzoin or Skin-Prep to the top of your patient's nose. When the benzoin or Skin-Prep feels tacky, place the tab end of the tape over it. Then, spiral one end of the tape around the tube. Take the other end under the tube and secure it on top of your patient's nose.

Important: Never tape the tube to your patient's forehead. The resulting tension may cause a pressure sore in his nasal passage.

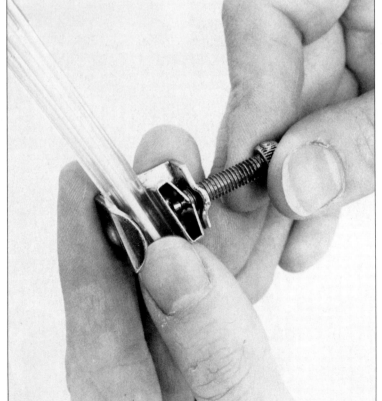

17 But, if your patient has a Levin-type tube in place, clamp it with a Hoffman clamp, as shown here. To keep it clean, cover the open end of the tube with gauze and secure it with a rubber band.

Suppose your patient complains of nausea. Leave the tube unclamped until the feeling subsides. Also, attach a drainage bag to provide an outlet for gastric contents.

18 To prevent the tube from dangling and possibly becoming dislodged, wrap a piece of adhesive tape around the end of the tubing and leave a tab. Then, using a safety pin, attach the tape tab to your patient's gown, just below his shoulder.

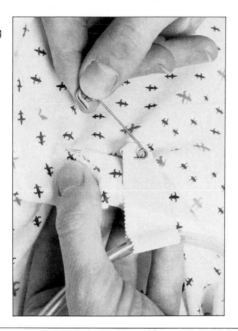

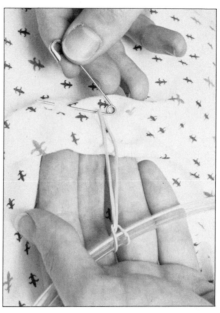

19 Or, loop a rubber band around the tube in a slipknot, as shown here. Pin the rubber band to your patient's gown.

Remember to make your patient as comfortable as possible. To minimize nasal irritation, place a small amount of water-soluble lubricant in each nostril. Prevent pressure sores by checking regularly to make sure the tubing's positioned comfortably. Also, provide good mouth care.

Document the entire insertion procedure in your nurses' notes.

Inserting a small feeding tube

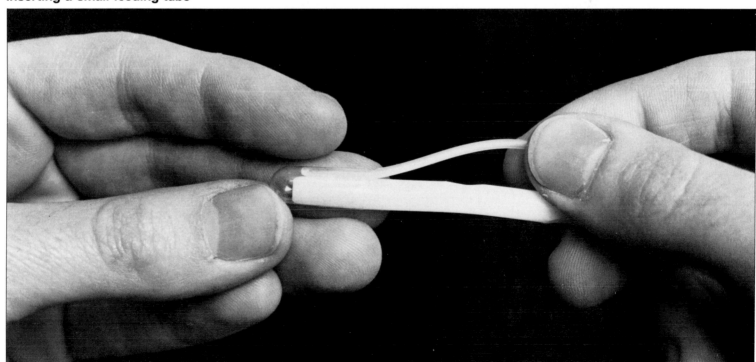

Are you caring for a patient who'll be tube feeding over a long time period? Most likely, the doctor will want you to insert a smaller feeding tube. Because the tube's smaller, your patient will find it less irritating than a regular size nasogastric (NG) tube.

To insert a smaller tube, first wedge the ends of a regular NG tube and the smaller feeding tube into half of a gelatin capsule, as shown in the photo above. Then, using the NG tube insertion guidelines, insert both tubes into your patient's stomach. Check tube placement, as explained on page 52.

When the tubes reach your patient's stomach, use tape to secure the outside ends to your patient's nose. Then, with a bulb syringe, inject about 30 ml of tap water into the NG tube, dissolving the gelatin capsule. Wait about 30 minutes, and untape the tubes.

Slowly withdraw the NG tube. Then, retape the tube to your patient's nose. Clamp the tube, or begin feedings, as ordered.

Document the procedure in your nurses' notes.

Nasogastric tube care

Checking tube placement

1 *Let's suppose you've just inserted a nasogastric (NG) tube. You'll want to make sure the
tube's in your patient's stomach, not his trachea,
before completing the procedure. To do this,
use two of the tests described below. If any of
your test results suggest that the tube's in your
patient's bronchus or trachea, withdraw the tube
immediately and try again.* Important: *Be especially careful about tube placement if your patient's
unconscious.*

The first two tests described here are the most
reliable methods to confirm tube placement.

Here's the first test: Attach a bulb or piston
syringe to the end of the tube and try to aspirate
gastric fluid, as shown here. If you can't withdraw
any fluid, the tube may be pressed against the
stomach wall, curled in the stomach, or not inserted far enough. In this case, reposition the tube
slightly and try again. If you still can't aspirate
gastric fluid, the tube may be in your patient's
bronchus.

Note: Even if you can aspirate gastric fluid,
don't assume the tube's properly placed. Your
patient may have gastric fluid in his lungs if he's
recently vomited and aspirated the vomitus.

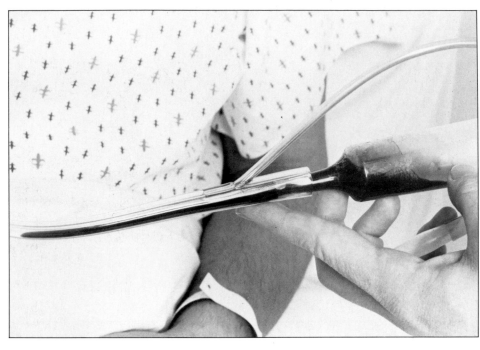

2 Then, try this second
test. Place a stetho-
scope over your patient's
stomach. Attach a bulb
syringe to the tube and inject
some air (about 30 cc) into
the tube. Then, as the nurse
is doing here, listen for air
entering the stomach
(a swooshing or gurgling
sound). Silence will indicate
that you haven't injected
air into the stomach, but into
your patient's bronchus or
esophagus.

Now, let's discuss some
other tests you can use.

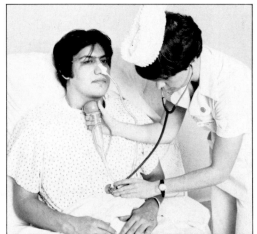

3 Hold the end of the
tube to your ear. You
shouldn't hear anything if the
tube's in your patient's stomach. If it's in his bronchus,
you'll hear crackling noises
and feel air coming from
the tube.

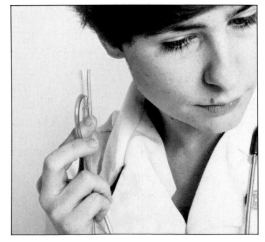

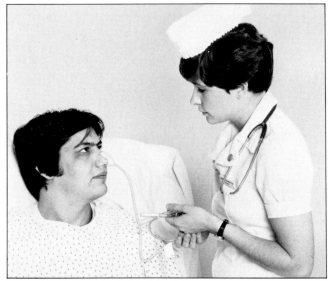

4 Or, try this test: Ask your conscious patient to hum. If
he can't, the tube may be in his trachea, separating
his vocal cords.

Note: Some nurses check for correct tube placement by
placing the end of the tube in a glass of water and
watching for air bubbles as the patient exhales. We don't
recommend this method because it's dangerous. If the
tube's in your patient's bronchus, he could aspirate water
as he inhales.

When at least *two* of these tests have verified correct
tube placement in your patient's stomach, advance the tube
or tape the tube in place and begin administering fluid
through the tube.

Important: If a test result raises any doubts, confirm
exact tube placement with an X-ray.

Administering a continuous drip tube feeding

1 *If the doctor wants your patient to receive a continuous feeding through her nasogastric (NG) tube, he'll ask you to set it up. Do you know how? This photostory will show you.*

Begin by assembling the equipment: feeding bag and tubing (we're using a Keofeed® enteric feeding bag and drip chamber tubing assembly), feeding solution as ordered, irrigating set with bulb syringe and water, stethoscope, glass of water, and bed-saver pad. You'll also need an I.V. pole.

Note: Tube feedings can also be given through an intestinal tube.

Make sure the feeding solution's at room temperature to prevent cramps and diarrhea. Explain the procedure to your patient, whether or not she's conscious.

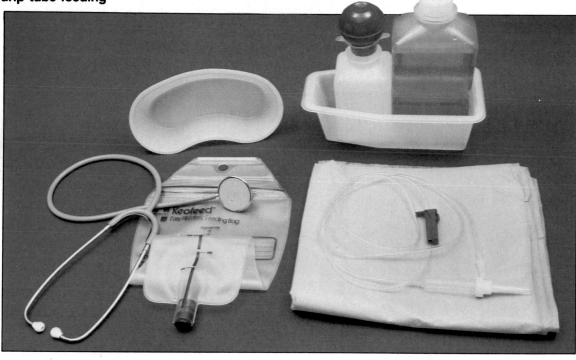

2 Place your patient in a semi-Fowler's position. Cover her gown with a bed-saver pad to keep it clean.

Now, confirm her tube's position, as explained on page 52.

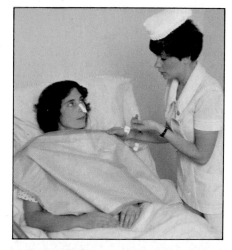

3 Close the roller clamp on the tubing. Then, remove the spike's protective cap. Firmly insert the spike into the Keofeed bag, as shown here.

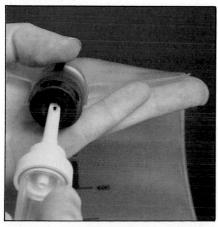

4 Now, hang the bag on the I.V. pole. Pour the proper amount of feeding solution into the bag.

Note: If this is your patient's first tube feeding, use water instead of feeding solution. On subsequent feedings, add feeding solution to the water in gradual amounts, until the patient's getting full-strength solution.

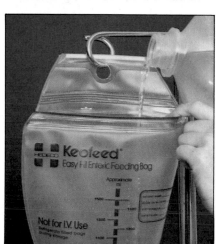

5 To seal the bag, apply pressure as you slide your fingers from one side of it to the other.

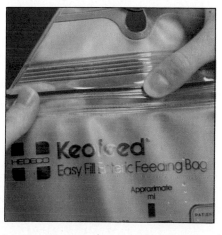
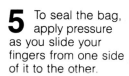

Nasogastric tube care

Administering a continuous drip tube feeding continued

6 Next, squeeze the drip chamber until it's half full of feeding solution. Hold the end of the tube over a basin or wastebasket. Then, open the roller clamp so the solution fills the tube. Close the clamp.

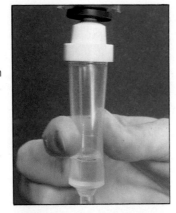

7 Now, attach your patient's NG tube to the feeding tube, as shown here. Tape both tubes together securely.

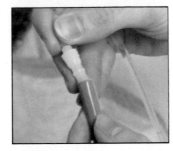

8 Open the roller clamp. Adjust the flow rate as ordered. (This tubing delivers about 20 drops per ml.)

Note: As you probably know, you can use a volumetric pump to regulate the feeding flow.

During the infusion, check your patient frequently to determine how she's tolerating the procedure, and to make sure her feeding tube remains properly positioned.

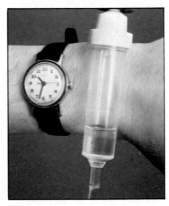

9 When the solution's infused, do one of the following, as ordered: pour in additional feeding solution; rinse and fill the bag with warm water, and infuse; or disconnect the tubing if the feeding's completed.

When the feeding's completed, use a bulb syringe and 30 to 50 ml water to clear your patient's tubing, to prevent clogging. Then, rinse the Keofeed bag and tube, and store them in a clean area until the next feeding.

Document the procedure in your nurses' notes.

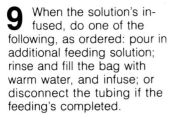
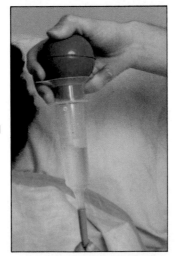

How to use a Ross gavage feeding set

1 *In this photostory, you'll see how to administer an Ensure tube feeding with a Ross gavage feeding set.*

To do this properly, you'll need to gather the necessary equipment: Ross gavage feeding set (includes suspension bag and tubing), Ensure feeding solution (at room temperature), bed-saver pad, towel, emesis basin, irrigating set with water and bulb syringe, and stethoscope. You'll also need an I.V. pole.

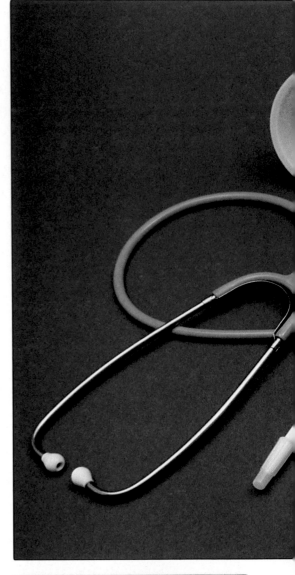

2 Now, examine the Ensure bottle. If you see any of the following, a broken seal, hairline cracks in the bottle, solution inconsistency, or past due expiration date, discard the bottle.

[Inset] But, if everything's okay, shake the bottle well to mix the solution thoroughly. Then, place the Ensure bottle into the suspension bag, as shown here. Uncap the bottle. If the bottle has never been opened, you'll hear a loud click.

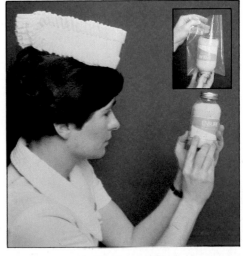

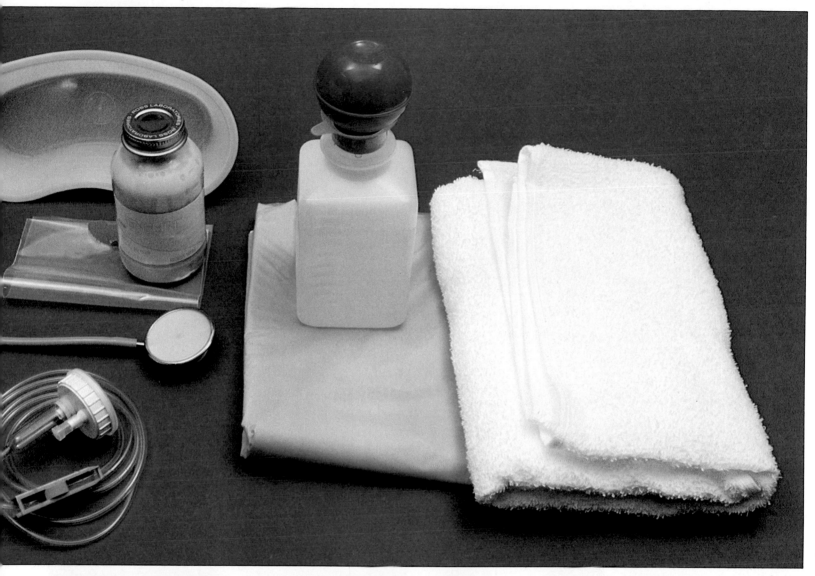

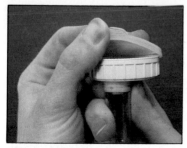

3 Now, snap off the overcap from the feeding set.

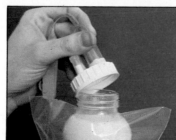

4 Screw the feeding cap onto the bottle. Close the flow regulator.
  Hang the suspension bag with the bottle inverted on the I.V. pole.

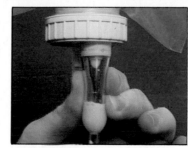

5 Squeeze the drip chamber until it's half full.
  Then, remove the cap from the end of the tube. To keep the cap from becoming contaminated, set it down with the open end up, or hold it, taking care not to touch the inside.

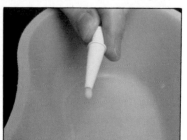

6 Hold the end of the tube over the emesis basin. Open the flow regulator and flush the line.
  Then, clamp the tube and replace the protective cap. Make sure the tubing is free of twists and obstructions.

Nasogastric tube care

How to use a Ross gavage feeding set continued

7 Now, have your patient sit in a semi-Fowler's position. Protect her bed linens and gown with the towel and bed-saver pad. Explain the procedure to her. Then, before proceeding further, check the position of her nasogastric (NG) tube using the tests described on page 52.

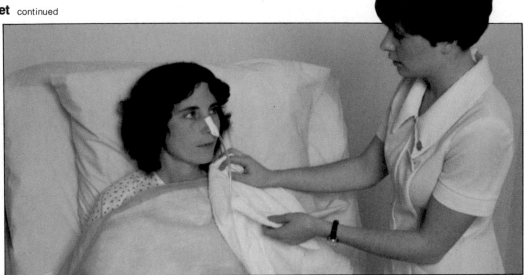

8 Next, connect the tubing to your patient's NG tube. Tape the connection together securely, as shown here.

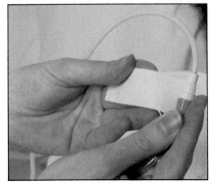

9 Use the roller clamp to adjust the flow rate, as ordered. As you may already know, the Ross gavage feeding set delivers 14 drops per ml.
Remember: The suspended bottle height and feeding tube size also affect the rate of infusion.
   Stay alert for any signs of patient intolerance to the feeding, such as nausea, cramps, diarrhea, or vomiting. Also, check your patient frequently to make sure the tube's in her stomach and taped securely.

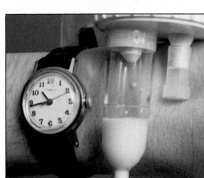

10 When the feeding bottle's empty, close the flow regulator. Then, depending on the doctor's orders, do one of three things: replace the empty bottle with a new one; or rinse the bottle, and fill it with the water needed to clear the tube.

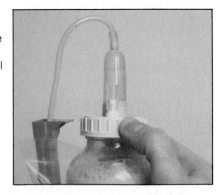

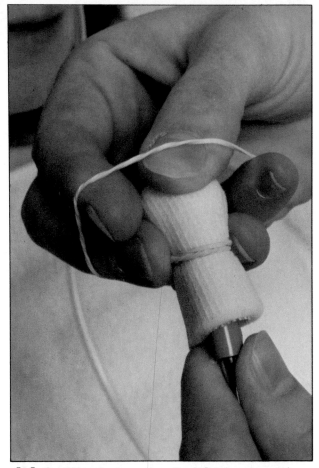

11 Or, if the doctor orders the NG tube clamped—and the feeding set discarded—flush the tube before you clamp it. Then wrap a gauze pad around the open end of the tube. Loop the rubber band around the gauze.
   Finally, document the entire procedure in your nurses' notes.

Administering an intermittent tube feeding

1 *Caring for a patient with a nasogastric (NG) tube? If so, you may have to administer intermittent tube feedings. Here's how:*

First, gather the equipment you'll need: irrigation set with bulb syringe (you can substitute a 50 cc piston syringe or a small funnel), stethoscope, towel or bed-saver pad, water to flush the tube, Hoffman clamp, tube feeding solution (as ordered), emesis basin, and measuring cup. Make sure the feeding solution is at room temperature. If it's too cold, your patient may develop stomach cramps, nausea, vomiting, or diarrhea.

Now, explain the procedure to your patient. Then, help him to a sitting position. Protect his gown with a bed-saver pad or towel, and place the emesis basin on his lap.

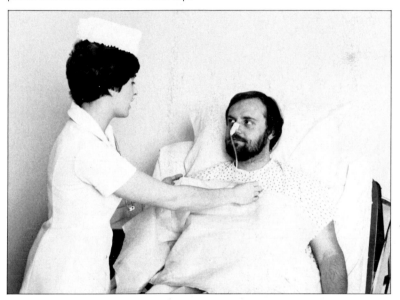

2 Unpin the NG tube from your patient's gown. Then, to prevent fluid reflux, hold the end of the tube above your patient's mouth and unclamp the tube. Remove the gauze from the end of the tube. Check tube placement by using at least two of the tests described on page 52.

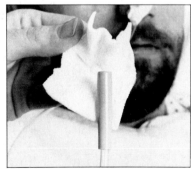

3 Before you begin the feeding, you'll aspirate your patient's gastric contents. Doing so enables you to check tube placement and patency, and helps you determine if his GI system is absorbing the feeding properly.

Attach the bulb syringe to the tube. To make aspiration easier, lower the syringe to just above his stomach level. Gently aspirate all his stomach contents. Remove the syringe, and place the end of the tube in an emesis basin.

4 Pour the aspirated gastric contents into a clean measuring cup. Are the contents more than half the volume of the previous feeding? If so, check with the doctor before proceeding. The tube feeding volume may be too great or your patient's GI system may not be absorbing the solution properly.

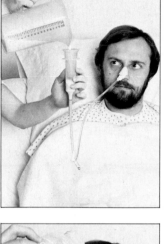

Next, remove the bulb from the bulb syringe and attach the syringe barrel to the NG tube. Hold the tube at your patient's head level. Pour the aspirated contents into the syringe, as the nurse is doing here. Let gravity carry the fluid back into your patient's stomach.

5 Now, as you hold the syringe at your patient's head level, slowly pour the prescribed feeding solution into the syringe. Let the feeding flow through the tube by gravity.

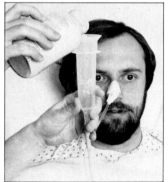

What if your patient complains of nausea, cramps, or a feeling of fullness? The solution may be infusing too rapidly. To control the infusion rate, raise or lower the level of the syringe.

Important: Never force the feeding down the tube.

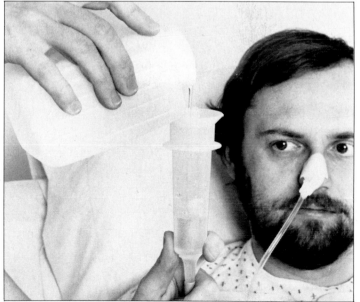

6 After you've infused the solution, flush your patient's tube with 30 ml of water, as shown here. Flushing clears the feeding solution from the ports at the end of the tube and prevents clogging.

Nasogastric tube care

Administering an intermittent tube feeding continued

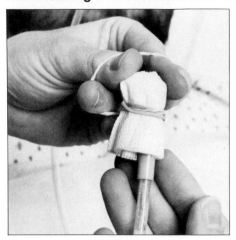

7 At this point, remove the syringe and clamp the tube. Place a gauze pad over the end of the tube and secure it with a rubber band. Then, pin the tube to your patient's gown. But, if your patient complains of nausea, leave the tube open until the feeling subsides.

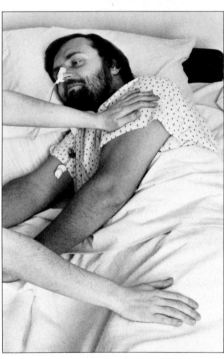

8 Ask your patient to remain in a sitting position for about 30 minutes. Doing so prevents vomiting and aspiration of the feeding. If he's uncomfortable sitting, place him in a right side-lying position with the head of the bed partially elevated, as shown here.

Suppose your patient develops diarrhea due to the solution's high osmolality. In this case, ask the doctor if you can give your patient smaller, more frequent feedings; change the type of tube feeding; or switch to a continuous drip method of tube feeding.

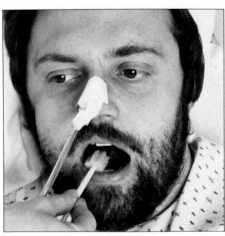

9 Now, wash and dry the syringe and return it to the container. Keep the irrigation set at your patient's bedside so it's ready for the next feeding. In addition, replace the entire irrigation set every 24 hours to minimize the chance of infection.

Provide good mouth care to keep your patient comfortable and prevent mouth ulcerations. Also, lubricate his nostrils to minimize irritation.

Finally, document the procedure in your nurses' notes.

Learning about gastric analysis

How does analyzing your patient's gastric secretions help the doctor assess your patient's condition? As you probably know, gastric analysis tells the doctor the volume and content of your patient's stomach secretions. When your patient's prepared properly, each of the three gastric tests tells you how much acid the stomach's producing, under three different circumstances. Two of the tests, basal analysis and stimulation analysis (which can be performed simultaneously), are performed to measure your patient's hydrochloric acid secretion. The third, hypoglycemic analysis (Hollander test), is usually performed to test the effectiveness of a vagotomy when that surgery has been done to reduce your patient's gastric acid secretion.

To prepare your patient for gastric analysis, follow these guidelines:
• Explain the procedure to your patient. Answer all his questions and reassure him.
• During the procedure, encourage your patient to expectorate excess saliva. Swallowing saliva may affect his gastric acidity level.
• Withhold anticholinergic drugs for 24 to 48 hours before testing, as ordered. As you know, anticholinergics reduce the GI tract's motility. Withholding these drugs encourages normal gastric secretion.
• Withhold all foods and fluids for 10 to 14 hours before testing. Otherwise, the results of the gastric analysis may not be accurate.
• On the morning of the test, make sure your patient has a properly positioned nasogastric (NG) tube in place. If he doesn't, insert one as described on pages 46 to 51.
• While you collect each specimen, have your patient assume each of these positions: sitting upright; sitting slightly forward; left side-lying (Sims'); right side-lying; and supine. Doing so allows for complete gastric suctioning.
• After withdrawing a *residual* specimen (complete stomach contents), test its acidity, using indicator dye (such as Töpfer's reagent), indicator paper, or a pH meter.
• As you perform each test, note the specimen's appearance. Notify the doctor if you see any of the following: any undigested food (may indicate gastric stasis or pyloric obstruction); fecal odor (may indicate neoplasm, gastric fistula, or intestinal obstruction); gross blood (may indicate an ulcerating lesion); or streaks of blood (may indicate trauma from NG tube insertion).
• After every test, label each specimen, and send it to the lab. In addition to evaluating the test results showing specimen volume and content, the doctor may also order cytologic studies and enzyme analysis. Indicate this on the lab slip.

Then, remove, clamp, or attach the NG tube to intermittent low suction, as ordered.

For details on each of the three tests, see the chart on the following page.

How to obtain specimens for gastric analysis

Type of analysis: Basal

Purpose: To determine the volume and content of your patient's normal gastric secretion without stimuli.

Nursing action:
• Using a bulb syringe, aspirate all of your patient's gastric contents into a specimen container. Label the specimen with your patient's name, his hospital identification number, and amount, date and time of collection. Remember, always mark the first specimen *residual contents.* Test the specimen's acidity.
• After 30 minutes, take another specimen. Label, as described above. Mark this specimen *basal contents* No. 1.
• Wait 15 minutes and take four more specimens, 15 minutes apart. Label as described above. Mark each *basal contents,* and 2, 3, 4, 5, accordingly.
• When you're finished, send the gastric specimens to the lab for analysis, as ordered. Then, remove the NG tube, clamp it, or attach it to intermittent low suction, as ordered.

Test results:
• Normal lab values are 2.0 ± 1.8 mEq/hr for females and 3.0 ± 2.0 mEq/hr for males.
• Marked increase in gastric secretion throughout this test may indicate Zollinger-Ellison syndrome (results of stimulation analysis necessary for confirmation).
• Absence of hydrochloric acid in gastric secretions may indicate pernicious anemia, or carcinoma.
• Excessive gastric secretions may indicate duodenal ulcer.

Type of analysis: Stimulation

Purpose: To determine the volume and content of your patient's gastric secretion after it has been stimulated with betazole hydrochloride (Histalog*) or pentagastrin (Peptavlon*).

Nursing action:
• Using a bulb syringe, aspirate all your patient's gastric contents into a specimen container. Label the specimen with your patient's name, his hospital identification number, and amount, date, and time of collection. Mark the first specimen *residual contents* and test the specimen's acidity.
• Wait 15 minutes and take four specimens, 15 minutes apart. Label each as described above. Mark each specimen *basal contents,* and No. 1, 2, 3, 4, accordingly.
• Administer betazole hydrochloride (Histalog) or pentagastrin (Peptavlon) subcutaneously, as ordered, to stimulate gastric secretion.
• Wait 15 minutes and collect four more specimens, 15 minutes apart. Label each as described above. Mark each specimen *stimulated contents* and No. 1, 2, 3, 4, accordingly.
• When you're finished, send the gastric specimens to the lab for analysis, as ordered. Then, remove the NG tube, clamp it, or attach it to intermittent low suction, as ordered.

Test results:
• Normal lab values are 16 ± 5 mEq/hr for females and 23 ± 5 mEq/hr for males.
• If your patient has a gastric ulcer—confirmed by endoscopy or X-ray—little or no secretion after stimulation may suggest gastric carcinoma.
• If your patient has a confirmed duodenal ulcer, and marked increase in basal output with the stimulation output greater than basal output, suspect Zollinger-Ellison syndrome.

*Available in both the United States and in Canada

Type of analysis: Hypoglycemic (Hollander test)

Purpose: To determine effectiveness of vagotomy, after surgery.

Nursing action:
• Have a prefilled syringe of 50% dextrose in water at your patient's bedside in case he develops any signs of hypoglycemia: weakness, vertigo, tremors, unconsciousness, and convulsions. Also, start an I.V. with normal saline solution or prescribed fluid, as ordered. If hypoglycemia is severe, be ready to switch I.V. to 10% dextrose in water.
• Draw blood for fasting blood sugar level. Label specimen with patient's name, his hospital identification number, and amount, date, and time of collection.
• Take patient's blood pressure and pulse to establish a baseline reading.
• Using a bulb syringe, aspirate your patient's gastric contents into a specimen container. Label the specimen as before. Mark the first specimen *residual contents.* Always test the specimen's acidity.
• Wait 15 minutes and collect four specimens, 15 minutes apart. Label each as described above. Mark each specimen *basal contents* and No. 1, 2, 3, 4 accordingly.
• Administer I.V. insulin, as ordered by the doctor.
• Then, taking one every 15 minutes, collect six more specimens. Label each specimen as described above. Mark each *stimulation specimen* and No. 5, 6, 7, 8, 9, 10, accordingly. In addition, check patient's blood pressure and pulse every 15 minutes. About 30 minutes after the insulin injection, draw blood for blood sugar level. Label as before and send to lab.
• After 15 minutes, draw another blood sample for blood sugar level. Label as before, and send to lab. At this point, the patient's blood sugar level should be at its lowest.
• About 1 hour after insulin injection, or when hypoglycemia symptoms disappear, draw another blood sample for blood sugar level. Label as before, and send to lab.

Test results:
• Normal lab values are 2.0 ± 1.8 mEq/hr for females and 3.0 ± 2.0 mEq/hr for males.
• If the surgery was successful, the patient will have no acid secretion after hypoglycemia has been induced.

Nasogastric tube care

Common tube feeding solutions: How they differ

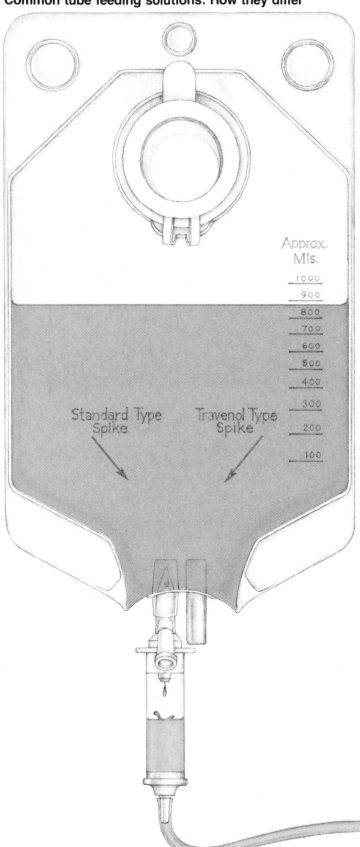

Approx. Mls.

1000
900
800
700
600
500
400
300
200
100

Standard Type Spike

Travenol Type Spike

Solution

Ensure® (Ross)
Provides patient with nutritionally complete diet. Contains 1 calorie per ml liquid, and low levels of sodium, potassium, cholesterol, and chloride. Solution is lactose-free.

Ensure® Plus (Ross)
Provides high caloric content, complete nutrition for a patient with intact GI system. Contains 1.5 calories per ml liquid, and is lactose-free.

Osmolite®
Provides nutrition for patients unable to tolerate other brands of tube feeding solutions. Contains medium chain triglycerides (MCT) as fats. Solution is lactose-free.

Precision LR Diet® (Doyle)
Provides patient with a nutritionally complete diet; low in residue and fat. Contains no lactose, gluten, cholesterol, or Vitamin K. Protein is egg albumin.

Precision Isotonic Diet® (Doyle)
Provides patient with a nutritionally complete diet that's low in residue and sodium. Contains no lactose, cholesterol, purine or gluten. Protein source is egg albumin.

Vital® (Ross)
Provides patient with a nutritionally complete diet that is low in lactose and residue. Protein source is peptides and free amino acids.

Amin-Aid® (McGaw)
Provides patient with essential amino acids and nonprotein calories that he requires in order to use accumulated urea nitrogen for protein synthesis. Contains low levels of sodium, potassium, calcium, and magnesium. Solution has no fiber or vitamins. Use only under medical supervision for a patient with renal insufficiency.

Controlyte® (Doyle)
Provides patient with controlled protein and low levels of electrolytes. Used only under medical supervision for a patient with severe liver disease, hepatic coma, or renal failure.

Advantages	Disadvantages
• Ready to use • May also be used as an oral food supplement. • Low cost per serving	• Contraindicated for patients with GI absorption disorders • Caloric content too low for some patients • Patient may develop signs of GI sensitivity to this feeding; for example, diarrhea, vomiting, and cramps.
• Ready to use • May also be used as an oral food supplement. • Low cost per serving • Recommended for patients who need high caloric nutrition, but can't tolerate increased fluid intake	• Patient may develop signs of GI sensitivity to this feeding; for example, diarrhea, vomiting, and cramps.
• Ready to use • May also be used as an oral food supplement. • Low cost per serving • Rapidly absorbed in upper GI tract • Recommended for patients with GI absorption disorders • Low osmolality	• Patient may develop signs of GI sensitivity to this feeding; for example, diarrhea, vomiting, and cramps.
• Easy to mix • May also be used as an oral food supplement. • Moderate cost per serving • Rapidly absorbed in upper GI tract • Recommended for patients with chronic diarrhea or recent bowel surgery	• Usually not used as an initial tube feeding • Patient may develop signs of GI sensitivity to feeding; for example, vomiting, diarrhea, and cramps. • Egg albumin may cause allergic reaction in some patients.
• May also be given as an oral food supplement. • Moderate cost per serving • Recommended for patient with GI disorders, pre- and postop patients, and patients who haven't ingested food for several weeks • Low osmolality	• Needs blending before administration. • Contraindicated for patients with impaired ability to utilize carbohydrates • Patient may develop signs of GI sensitivity to this feeding; for example, diarrhea, vomiting, and cramps. • Egg albumin may cause allergic reaction in some patients.
• May be given as an oral supplement. • Moderate cost per serving • Rapidly absorbed in upper GI tract • Recommended for a patient needing hydrolized diets; or, for a patient with long-term tube feedings	• Feeding separates after mixing. • Patient may develop signs of GI sensitivity to feeding; for example, diarrhea, vomiting, and cramps.
• Lowers BUN levels	• More successful as an oral supplement • Very high cost per serving • Patient may develop signs of GI sensitivity to feeding; for example, vomiting, diarrhea, and cramps. • Patient must be closely monitored because of low mineral and electrolyte content.
• After mixing, feeding may be refrigerated until used. • May be used as a food supplement. • Moderate cost per serving	• Patient may develop signs of GI sensitivity to feeding; for example, vomiting, diarrhea, and cramps. • Contains no vitamins.

Nasogastric tube care

Assessing tube-feeding effectiveness

Is your patient receiving feeding solution through a nasogastric (NG) tube? If so, determine the solution's effectiveness by assessing your patient routinely and watching for the following signs and symptoms:

• *vomiting.* May indicate the solution is contaminated, the infusion rate's too rapid, the patient's sensitive to the solution, or the patient has an intestinal obstruction.

• *diarrhea.* May indicate the solution is contaminated, the infusion rate's too rapid, or the solution's too cold.

• *constipation.* May indicate the patient is sensitive to the solution or is dehydrated.

• *decreased urine output, elevated temperature, soft and sunken eyeballs, skin coolness and blanching, and increased pulse rate.* May indicate the patient is dehydrated or has a severe bacterial infection.

• *swelling or edema, especially in legs or sacral area; rapid weight gain.* May indicate patient is retaining fluid.

If you note any of the above (or your patient complains of nausea or a feeling of fullness), notify the doctor. Depending on your observations, he may want you to: increase or decrease the infusion rate; warm, change, or discontinue the solution; or, supplement the solution with increased fluid, via NG tube or by I.V.

Of course, whenever your patient is receiving a tube feeding, you must:

• check NG tube placement before each feeding.

• take vital signs at least once every 4 hours.

• draw blood for serum electrolyte testing, as ordered.

• provide good mouth and nose care.

• weigh him on the same scale and at the same time each day.

• keep accurate fluid intake and output records.

• document everything in your nurses' notes.

How to irrigate a nasogastric tube

1 *Let's suppose you've just given a tube feeding. Now, you're ready to irrigate the tube. As you know, you'll irrigate a nasogastric (NG) tube once every 2 hours, or as ordered, to prevent clogging. Here's how:*

Start by obtaining an irrigation set; irrigation solution, as ordered (usually normal saline solution or tap water); towel or bed-saver pad; emesis basin; stethoscope; and piston syringe (optional).

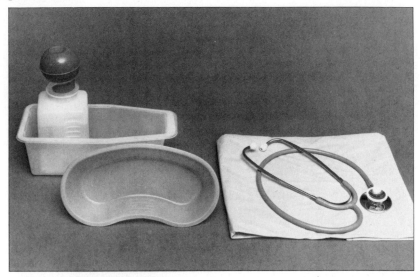

2 Explain the irrigating procedure to your patient. Then, raise the head of his bed so he's sitting upright. Doing so helps prevent fluid reflux, which could lead to aspiration.

Cover his gown with a towel or bed-saver pad. Make sure the NG tube is properly secured to his nose.

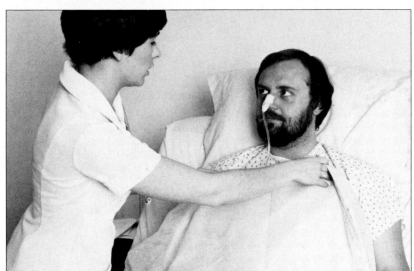

3 Unclamp your patient's tube. Check the tube's position in your patient's stomach, using two of the tests explained on page 52.

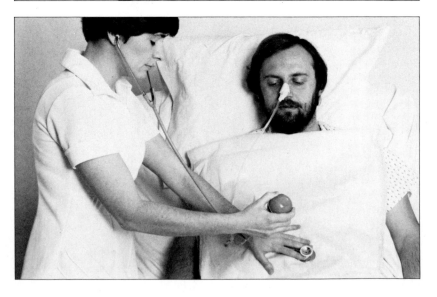

4 Remove the bulb from the syringe. Then, attach the syringe to the NG tube. Pour 30 ml of irrigating solution into a bulb syringe. Let gravity carry the solution to your patient's stomach.

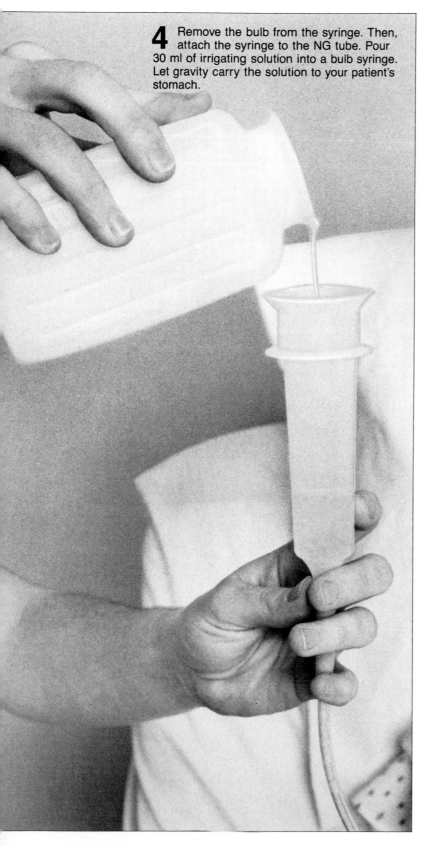

5 Suppose the solution doesn't flow down the tube. Attach the bulb to the syringe. Then, compress the bulb firmly, pushing the fluid through the tube.

Note: Be sure to apply enough pressure to push the solution through the tube.

Now, gently withdraw the solution, using the bulb syringe, as shown here. If you have difficulty, inject 20 cc of air and try again. Suppose you still can't withdraw the solution. Try repositioning the tube, or your patient. Either may move the end of the tube away from his stomach wall, allowing for fluid aspiration. If you continue having trouble, reconnect the tube to intermittent low suction and notify the doctor.

Caution: Never aspirate forcefully. If the tube is against the gastric mucosa, vigorous pulling may cause superficial erosions.

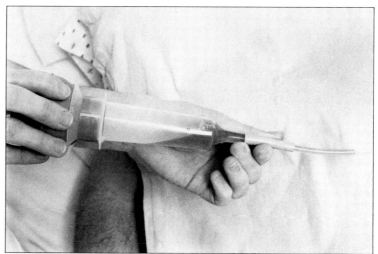

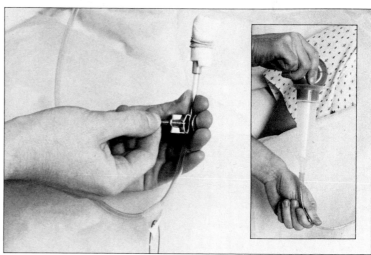

6 Has the doctor ordered an irrigation with more than 30 ml of solution? If so, continue the irrigation procedure, instilling 30 ml at a time until you've administered the prescribed amount.

When you've finished irrigating, reconnect your patient's tube to intermittent low suction, or clamp it, as ordered.

[Inset] Suppose your patient has a Salem Sump® tube. After reconnecting the tube to suction, you'll inject the vent lumen with air. Doing so ensures the vent lumen's patency for sump action.

Finally, document the procedure in your nurses' notes.

Nasogastric tube care

How to perform gastric lavage

1 *Consider this situation: James Welsh, a 30-year-old chemist, has just been admitted to the hospital with a phenobarbital overdose. The doctor instructs you to perform a gastric lavage. Here's what to do:*

First, gather the equipment: a large irrigating or bulb syringe; 1,200 to 5,000 ml tap water or normal saline solution (100 ml if your patient's a child); two basins; suctioning machine; and the appropriate antidote, as ordered.

Explain the procedure to your patient. Then, insert a nasogastric (NG) tube, as described on pages 46 to 51.

Caution: Never perform a gastric lavage if your patient's taken a corrosive agent, such as lye, ammonia, or mineral acids. Instead, neutralize the agent with the proper antidote, and follow the doctor's instructions.

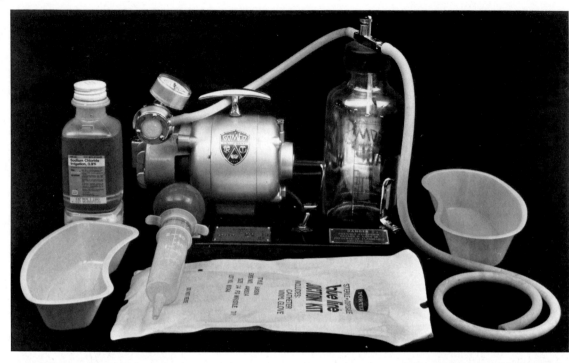

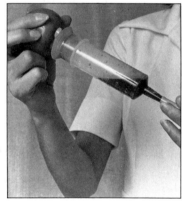

2 Now, place Mr. Welsh in a high Fowler's position (or as ordered by the doctor).

Note: If your patient's combative and tries to pull out his NG tube, you may need to get a doctor's order to restrain him.

Make sure the NG tube's positioned properly. (For information on checking tube placement, see page 52.) Then, attach the syringe to the tube. Aspirate your patient's stomach contents and empty them into a basin. Put the basin aside. Later, you'll send a labeled container of stomach contents to the lab for analysis.

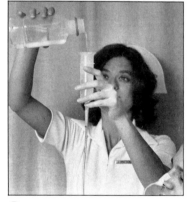

3 Remove the bulb from the syringe. Lift the end of the tube above Mr. Welsh's head. Then, pour about 500 ml (no more) of water or saline solution into the tube. Stay alert for signs of stomach overfilling, such as vomiting or distention.

If your patient starts to vomit, stop pouring the water *immediately* and turn his head to the side. Then, let the NG tube drain. Suction his mouth and trachea. Make sure his airway's open before proceeding.

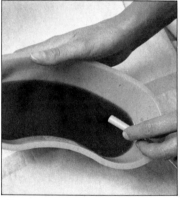

4 Now, place the remaining basin next to Mr. Welsh. Remove the syringe barrel from the tube and put the end of the tube into the basin. The gravitational pull will siphon your patient's stomach contents. Repeat this entire procedure at least 10 times, or until you withdraw clear fluid from his stomach.

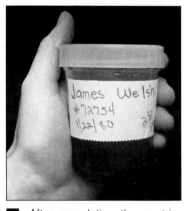

5 After completing the gastric lavage, do one of the following, as ordered: instill the correct antidote, close the tube with a temporary clamp, allow gravity to drain the tube, attach intermittent low suction, or remove the tube.

Important: If your hospital requires you to send aspirated stomach contents to the lab for analysis, be sure to pour them into a properly labeled container. In suspected drug overdose cases, check your hospital policy before discarding stomach contents.

Document your findings.

How to perform an iced gastric lavage

1 *The time is 2 a.m., you've just returned from your break, and 29-year-old Helen Johnson arrives in the emergency department (ED) suffering from an uncontrolled gastric hemorrhage. The doctor orders an iced gastric lavage stat. Here's how to proceed:*

Begin by gathering the necessary equipment: bulb syringe with solution container, basin filled with ice, 2 to 3 liters saline solution (the doctor may order iced tap water for a patient with a sodium restriction), an empty basin for return fluid, an emesis basin, a measuring cup, bed-saver pad, tissues, water-soluble lubricant, and a large-lumen gastric tube (size 36 to 40 French). In this photostory we're using a size 40 French Lavacuator II™ tube. You'll also need a suction machine with suction catheter.

Important: Don't use a gastric tube smaller than size 36 French or it may become clogged with blood clots.

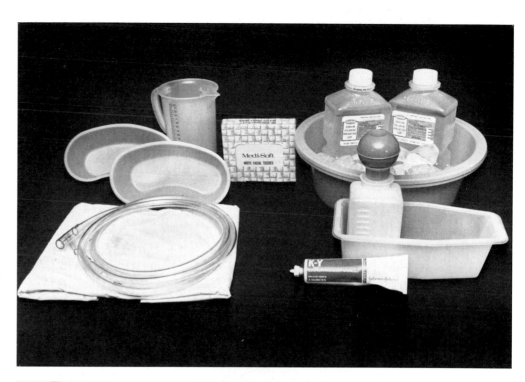

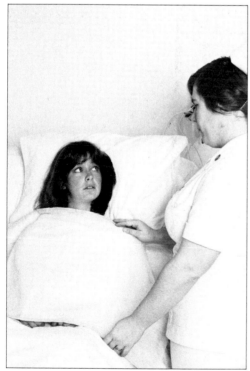

2 Explain the procedure to your patient. She'll probably be extremely anxious, so encourage her questions and reassure her. Put a blanket over her to keep her warm.

Chill the saline solution in a basin of ice. Then, pour the solution into the container.

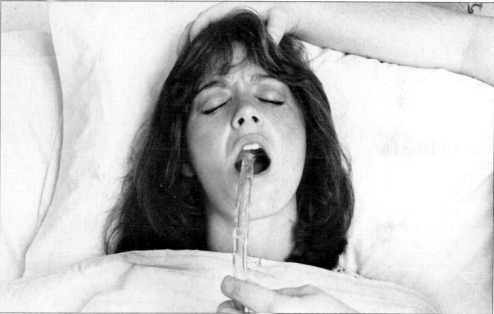

3 Now, you're ready to insert the gastric tube. To do this, place Ms. Johnson in a high Fowler's position and cover her gown with a bed-saver pad.

Important: If your patient doesn't exhibit a gag reflex, have a respiratory therapist or other trained professional insert an endotracheal tube prior to insertion of the gastric tube. This will ensure an open airway, and prevent aspiration. Be prepared to assist with the insertion.

Before you insert the gastric tube, lubricate the end of it with water-soluble lubricant. Then, insert the tube into your patient's mouth, toward her oropharynx.

Once the tube is in your patient's pharynx, pass the tube into her stomach. Check tube placement as explained on page 52.

Remember: When you insert a gastric tube orally, your patient can't sip water or chew ice chips.

Nasogastric tube care

How to perform an iced gastric lavage continued

4 When the tube's in place, lower the head of the bed to 15°.
Place Ms. Johnson in a left side-lying position, so the tube will lie along the greater curve of her stomach.

Suppose turning your patient onto her left side is contraindicated. Keep her in a high Fowler's position to prevent her from aspirating vomitus.

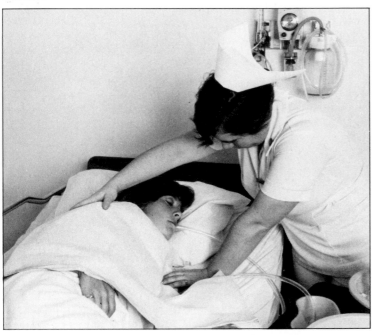

6 When you're sure the tube's properly placed, fill the syringe with 30 to 40 ml of the iced saline solution. Then, attach the syringe to the tube, and inject saline solution into the tube. Keep the tube as still as possible. Wait about 30 seconds.

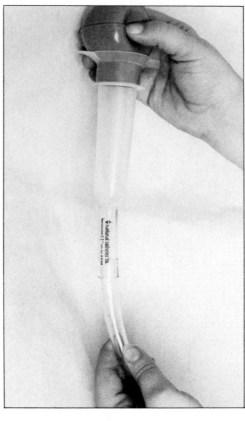

5 Now, attach a bulb syringe to the end of the tube, and try to aspirate gastric fluid. If no fluid can be withdrawn, clear the tube by injecting 20 cc of air. If you still get no return, try repositioning the tube. The tube may be positioned too high in the stomach, pressed against your patient's stomach mucosa, or curled.

Caution: Never aspirate gastric fluid forcefully. If the tube is against the stomach mucosa, you may cause tissue erosions.

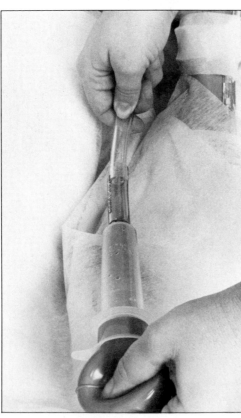

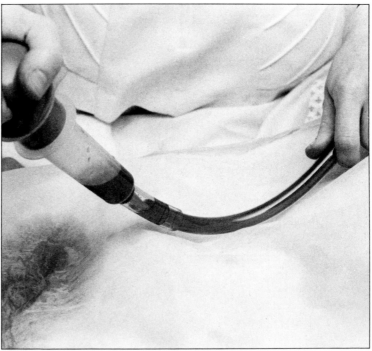

7 Now, withdraw the fluid into the syringe. If you're unable to withdraw fluid, allow the tube to drain into the emesis basin. Put the fluid into a container.

Continue to reassure your patient.

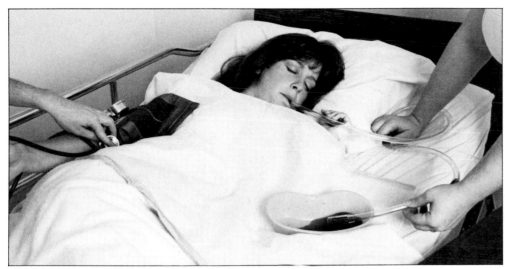

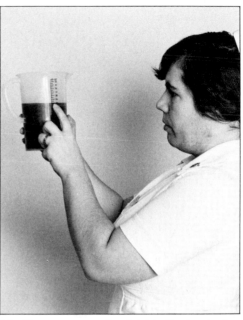

8 As you're performing the lavage, ask a coworker to closely monitor Ms. Johnson's blood pressure and pulse. Individually, the lavage procedure or uncontrolled gastric hemorrhaging can lead to hypothermia. In combination, the risk of lowered body temperature is even greater. As you know, hypothermia may precipitate cardiac arrhythmias.

Continue the lavage until the return fluid is clear (or as ordered). When you've completed the lavage, empty any remaining fluid from your patient's stomach. Then, tape the tube to her cheek, or remove and discard it, as ordered.

9 Now, measure the fluid in the basin. In your nurses' notes, document its color, amount and consistency. Also, document your patient's tolerance of the procedure.

Iced lavage: How to use a double-lumen gastric tube

You'll insert a double-lumen gastric tube when the doctor wants your patient to have a more rapid iced gastric lavage; such as in cases of massive, uncontrolled gastric hemorrhage. A double-lumen tube allows for faster infusion of the iced saline solution. Most double-lumen gastric tubes come in large sizes: 36 to 40 French. They're usually passed orally, but may be passed nasally, if ordered.

Whenever you perform an iced gastric lavage with a double-lumen tube, you'll attach intermittent low suction to the large port (see inset) as you instill the iced saline solution into the small port. In addition, remember to closely monitor your patient's vital signs and keep her as warm as possible.

Has the doctor ordered a continuous iced saline flow? If so, use a kangaroo feeding bag (the one shown here is made by Chesebrough-Pond's, Inc.) This two-chambered bag—with one chamber holding the ice and the other chamber holding the saline solution—makes the procedure quicker and easier.

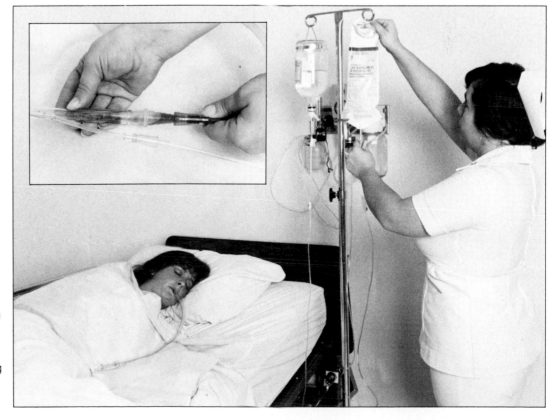

Nasogastric tube care

Caring for a patient with a GI hemorrhage

Michael Roth, a 48-year-old salesman, was admitted to the intensive care unit (ICU) with a bleeding duodenal ulcer. As you're taking his blood pressure, he suddenly begins vomiting large amounts of bright red blood. You suspect a massive GI hemorrhage.

To stop Mr. Roth's bleeding quickly and replace his lost blood, you and your coworkers will be working as a team, performing several procedures simultaneously. Do you know how to proceed? Check your skills using the information on these pages.

But remember, your patient's mental status is as important as his physical. Reassure him as much as possible. Explain each procedure to him as it's performed, even if he's unconscious. In addition, reassure your patient's family, and report to them frequently about his condition. Document all procedures in your nurses' notes.

Monitor Mr. Roth's vital signs until the bleeding's controlled; and make sure his airway's patent. Also watch him closely for signs of hypovolemic shock, which include: low blood pressure; cold, clammy skin; decreased urinary output; increased respiratory rate; restlessness; and diaphoresis. If you see any of these signs, or if your patient complains of dizziness or nausea, notify the doctor. Until properly typed and crossmatched blood's available, he may order Type O, Rh negative blood, or plasma administered intravenously.

Place your patient in a side-lying position, with his head slightly elevated. This position helps prevent aspirating of vomitus. Also, cover him with a blanket.

Prepare for nasogastric (NG) tube insertion by placing your patient in high Fowler's position, or as ordered.

Insert the tube as explained on pages 46 to 51. Then, attach the NG tube to intermittent low suction, as ordered. Note the color, amount, and consistency of the aspirated gastric contents.

Draw a blood sample for determining type and crossmatch, complete blood count (CBC), hemoglobin and hematocrit levels, and electrolyte balance. Also, obtain an arterial sample to determine blood gas measurements. Label the samples with your patient's name, his hospital identification number, the date, and time. Send the samples to the laboratory for immediate analysis.

Remember: Keep the arterial blood sample on ice to ensure accurate test results.

Administer oxygen at a flow rate of 2 to 4 liters via nasal cannula, as ordered. After the doctor gets the results from the arterial blood gas measurement, he'll adjust the O_2 flow rate accordingly.

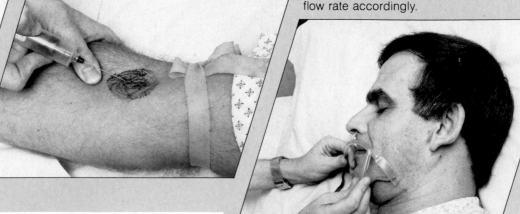

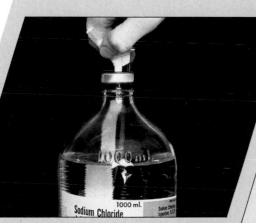

Start an I.V. infusion of normal saline solution, as ordered.

After your patient's blood is typed and cross-matched, begin a blood transfusion, as ordered. (See the NURSING PHOTOBOOK *Managing I.V. Therapy* for details.)

Watch Mr. Roth closely for any adverse reactions to the blood transfusion, such as diaphoresis, itching, or respiratory distress. If you see any, stop the transfusion and notify the doctor. Return the unused blood and tubing to the lab.

If after 15 minutes everything's okay, increase the I.V. infusion rate, as ordered.

Insert a Foley catheter, as ordered. (For insertion guidelines, see the NURSING PHOTOBOOK *Implementing Urologic Procedures*.) Then, collect and label a sterile urine specimen to send to the lab for analysis.

Attach the Foley catheter to a urine meter. Every hour, measure the amount of urine that's collected in the drainage chamber. In your notes, record the amount, color, and consistency of the urine. If Mr. Roth's urine output is less than 30 ml an hour, notify the doctor. He may want to increase the I.V. infusion rate.

When the bleeding's controlled, administer cimetidine (Tagamet*) I.V., as ordered, to keep it from recurring. Prepare your patient for upper GI endoscopy, as ordered, to locate the bleeding site. Doing so will help determine future treatment. Be prepared to assist the patient's doctor with the procedure, as needed.

If Mr. Roth's gastrointestinal bleeding remains uncontrolled, prepare him for surgery (gastric resection), as ordered by the doctor.

If the hemorrhage isn't self-limiting, get ready to perform iced gastric lavage. Insert a large gauge (36 to 40 French) gastric tube and begin the procedure, as ordered (for more information, see pages 65 and 66).

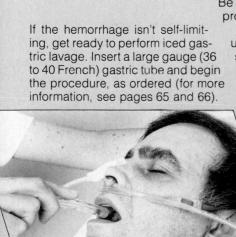

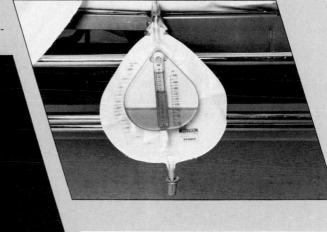

Nasogastric tube care

Removing a nasogastric tube

1 *Has the doctor asked you to remove your patient's nasogastric (NG) tube? If so, follow these steps:*

First, explain the procedure to your patient. Then place her in a high Fowler's position. Use a towel or bed-saver pad to protect her gown and bed linens from spills.

Then, unpin the tube from her gown. Remove the tape from her nose.

3 When the tube moves freely, inject 30 cc air into it, to clear out any remaining fluid. Then, reclamp the tube with a hemostat. Or, fold the tube in your hands, as shown in this photo. Both methods prevent fluid from entering your patient's lung while you remove the tube.

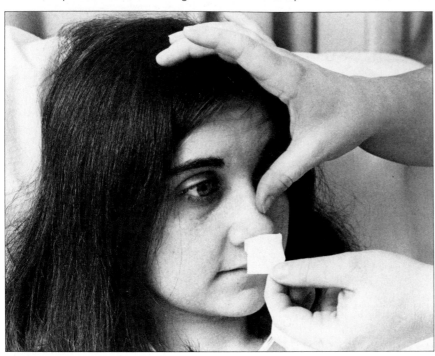

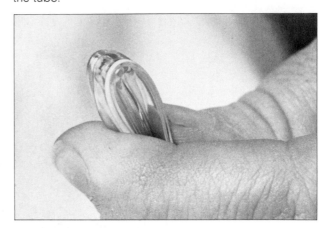

2 Gently rotate the tube to make sure it moves freely. If it doesn't, flush the tube with normal saline solution. To do this, remove the bulb from a bulb syringe and attach the syringe to the tube. Then, pour 30 ml of the solution into the syringe and unclamp the tube. Gravity will pull the solution down the tube.

Suppose the solution doesn't flow down the tube. Then, try irrigating the tube gently, as described on pages 62 to 63.

If you still can't rotate the tube, notify the doctor.

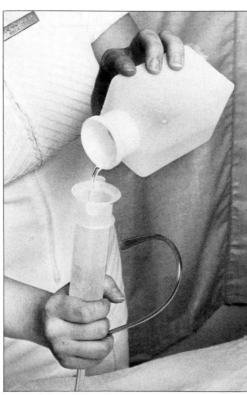

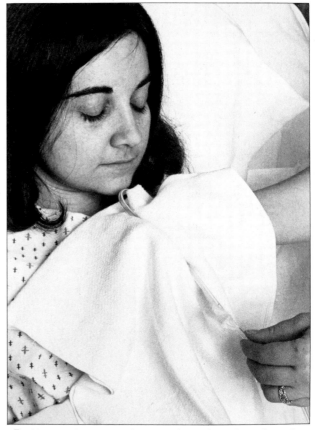

4 Now, ask your patient to take a deep breath and hold it as you quickly withdraw the tube. Then, place the tube on a towel, out of the patient's sight, if possible. When you've removed the tube, tell your patient to resume breathing. Give her the mouth care she'll need to feel comfortable.

Document the procedure in your nurses' notes.

Gastrostomy care

How adept are you at caring for a patient with a gastric resection? For example, suppose the doctor's inserted a Penrose drain at the incision site? Do you know how to protect your patient's skin from drainage? Can you identify the signs and symptoms of dumping syndrome? Do you know how to prevent or help control this condition?

And what about a patient with a gastrostomy tube? Can you change a gastrostomy dressing? Do you know how to administer a tube feeding via a gastrostomy tube? How to check a gastrostomy tube's patency?

If you're not sure, read the following pages. In them you'll find the answers to these important questions and much, much more.

How to administer a tube feeding via gastrostomy tube

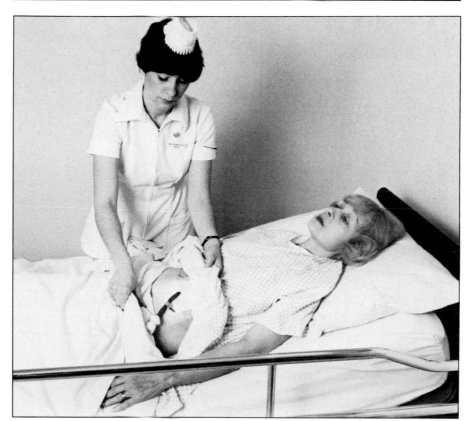

1 *You're caring for Jessica McCarran, a 65-year-old, retired bookkeeper who's just had a gastrostomy. During surgery, the doctor inserted a gastrostomy tube. Do you know how to administer a feeding through a gastrostomy tube? If you're unsure, follow these steps:*

Begin by gathering the equipment: bulb syringe (you can also use a piston syringe or funnel), prescribed tube feeding solution warmed to room temperature, 30 ml water to flush the tube, bed-saver pad or towel, 4"x4" gauze pads, and a rubber band.

2 Now, explain the procedure to Ms. McCarran. Then, expose her gastrostomy tube, as the nurse is doing here. Be sure to cover her with a blanket to keep her warm.

Gastrostomy care

How to administer a tube feeding via gastrostomy tube continued

3 Remove the gauze from the end of her gastrostomy tube, and unclamp the tube. Then, remove the bulb from the syringe. Attach the syringe to the tube, as shown here.

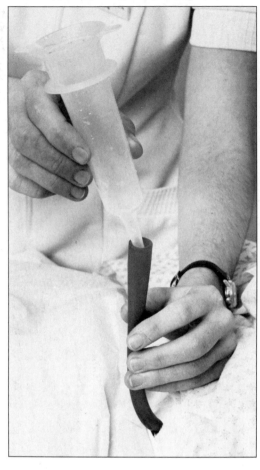

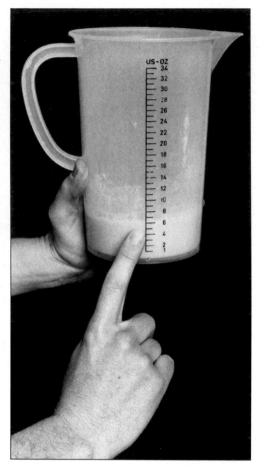

5 Then, measure and record the amount of aspirated contents. Pour the aspirated gastric contents back into her stomach, using the bulb syringe. Then, notify the doctor. Are the aspirated contents more than half of the last tube feeding? If so, the doctor may decrease the amount or frequency of your patient's feeding.

Then, try flushing the tube again. If the water still backs up, irrigate the tube, as explained on page 73.

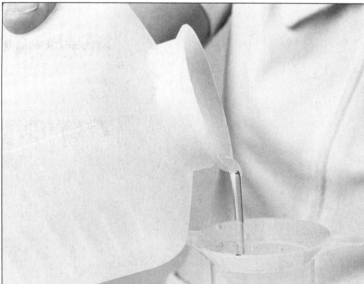

4 To test the tube's patency, flush it with 30 ml of water. If the water backs up, the tube may be clogged or solution from the last tube feeding may still be in Ms. McCarran's stomach.

Use a bulb syringe to aspirate your patient's stomach contents into a container.

6 When the tube's been completely flushed, hold the end 3" to 6" (7.6 to 15.2 cm) above your patient's stomach. Slowly pour the prescribed feeding solution into the tube, as the nurse is doing here. Allow the solution to flow through the tube by gravity.

Important: Never force feeding solution through the tube. Suppose the solution oozes out around the incision. Stop the procedure immediately, and notify the doctor. The tube may have pulled out of the stomach.

7 After you've infused all the feeding solution, flush out the tube with 30 to 50 ml water. Doing so will clear the tube and prevent clogging.

Hold the tube upright. Then, remove the syringe and clamp the tube with a Hoffman clamp, as shown here.

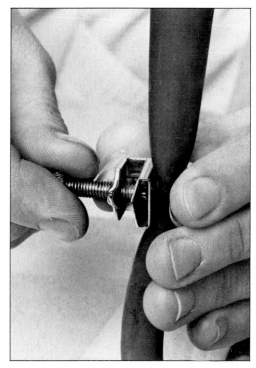

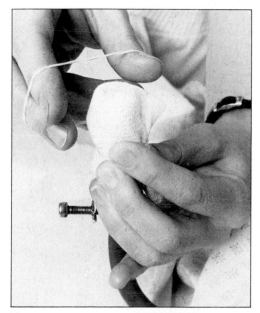

8 Next, place a 4"x4" gauze pad over the end of the tube. Secure the gauze with a rubber band, as shown. Document the procedure in your nurses' notes.

How to irrigate a gastrostomy tube

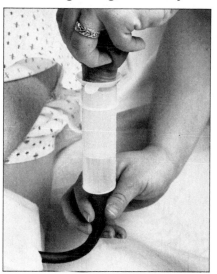

1 *In the previous photostory you learned how to check the patency of a gastrostomy tube. If the tube's clogged—and you've determined that the patient's stomach isn't distended—you must irrigate the tube. Make sure irrigating is okay with the doctor. Then, proceed as follows:*

First, remove the bulb from a bulb syringe. Attach the syringe filled with tap water or normal saline solution to the end of the gastrostomy tube. Pour 30 to 40 ml tap water or normal saline solution into the syringe. Then, replace the bulb, as shown here. Firmly compress the bulb. This should remove the blockage.

But, in some cases, you may need to compress the bulb several times.

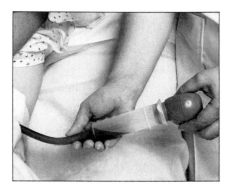

2 To determine if the irrigation was successful, remove the syringe from the tube and squeeze the bulb. This creates a vacuum.

Then, reattach the syringe to the tube and release the bulb, creating a suction. If the tube's patent, you'll aspirate gastric contents.

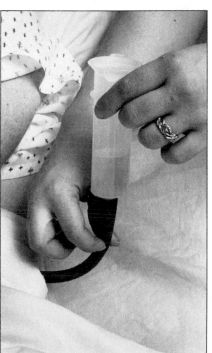

3 Suppose you still can't aspirate gastric contents. Repeat the irrigation. If you're still unsuccessful, reclamp the tube and notify the doctor.

Document the procedure in your nurses' notes.

Gastrostomy care

How to change a gastrostomy dressing

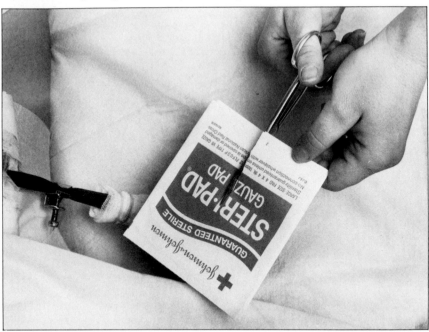

1 *Let's suppose you notice that your patient's gastrostomy dressing has become soiled. You'll want to change the dressing immediately to prevent skin excoriation and decrease the chance of infection.*

In this procedure, you'll use a precut sponge, if you have one. Or, make one by cutting a slit halfway through the middle of two unopened 4"x4" gauze pads, as the nurse is doing here.

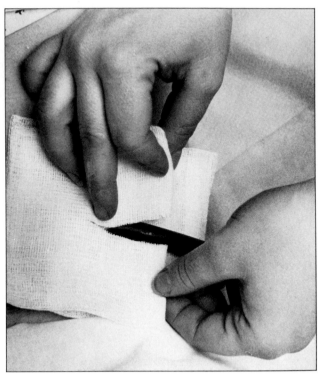

3 Remove the cut 4"x4" gauze pads from their wrappers. Fit them snugly around the tube with the slits overlapping, as shown in this photo.

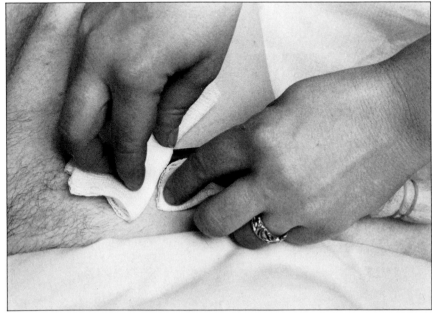

2 Now, remove the soiled dressing. Wash the skin around your patient's gastrostomy site with mild soap and warm water. Rinse and dry the skin thoroughly.

Then, closely examine the gastrostomy site for redness or swelling. If you see either, apply a skin barrier, such as karaya or Stomahesive, to the skin around the tube.

Note: If the sutures aren't holding the gastrostomy tube firmly in place, tape the tube securely to your patient's abdomen.

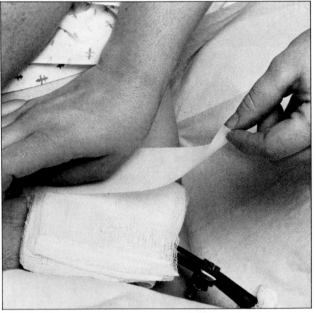

4 Next, cover these pads with an uncut 4"x4" gauze pad. Secure the entire dressing with two strips of 2"-wide, nonallergenic adhesive tape.

Remember: You must change the dressing on your patient's gastrostomy site at least once daily, or immediately if it becomes loose or soiled.

Document the dressing change in your nurses' notes.

Clinical management of a patient with a peptic ulcer

To care for a patient with a peptic ulcer, you must first examine the treatment program ordered by the doctor. Do you know how a peptic ulcer should be managed clinically? If you're unsure, read what follows:
• *Diet:* Rely on your patient to tell you which foods cause pain, and instruct him to avoid them. Also, tell him to avoid foods that are extremely hot or cold, as well as excessive use of caffeinic and alcoholic beverages.

Initially, he should eat six small meals daily. However, as healing progresses, he should gradually return to three reasonably sized meals a day.
• *Antacids:* As you probably know, antacids form the mainstay of ulcer treatment. Usually, a doctor selects an antacid according to its major component (such as aluminum or magnesium) and the patient's individual needs. For example, magaldrate (Riopan*) features a low sodium level and is suitable for elderly patients or patients with heart problems.

In early treatment, 15 to 30 ml (1 to 2 tablespoons) of liquid antacids, such as Gelusil*, Mylanta*, and Maalox, may be taken hourly, beginning 1 hour after breakfast and continuing until bedtime. Dosage frequency decreases as healing progresses, as ordered. In some cases, antacid dosages are alternated hourly with 30 ml of cream or milk to keep an alkaline substance in your patient's stomach. In such a case, you may administer antacids at 1, 2, and 3 p.m. and 30 ml of milk at 1:30, 2:30, and 3:30 p.m.
• *Anticholinergic drugs:* Used in combination with antacids, these drugs reduce the stomach's acid secretion and motor activity, allowing the antacids to stay in the stomach longer. In most cases, anticholinergic drugs are recommended for short-term therapy when pain is not relieved by antacids. Examples of anticholinergic drugs are atropine, and propantheline bromide (Pro-Banthine*).
• *Cimetidine (Tagamet*):* Cimetidine greatly reduces acid secretion in the stomach, relieving ulcer pain. Doses of 300 mg are given orally with each meal and at bedtime, for a maximum of 8 weeks. Because antacids interfere with cimetidine absorption, administer these drugs at least 1 hour apart, if possible. When healing occurs, cimetidine therapy is discontinued or the drug is given at night only.
• In addition to the above drugs, rest, sedatives, and tranquilizers can reduce your patient's anxiety and stress.

Knowing what's involved in the clinical management of an ulcer helps you effectively teach your patient. And, as you know, good patient teaching will help him prepare to continue his treatment outside the hospital, until his ulcer has healed.

Understanding dumping syndrome

How much do you know about dumping syndrome? If your patient's had a gastric resection, he may develop this condition after he begins eating solid foods again. Wondering why? Here's the reason. When the patient's pylorus is removed during surgery, hypertonic foods and liquids move from his stomach to his small intestine at an abnormally fast rate.

To accommodate this sudden onrush, large amounts of fluid are drawn from the patient's vascular system, overtaxing it. This brings on most of the signs and symptoms of dumping syndrome. These signs and symptoms include:
• abdominal cramping, diarrhea, and a feeling of fullness (from intestinal distention).
• weakness, faintness, dizziness, increased pulse rate, heart palpitations, and diaphoresis (from decreased plasma volume).

During your patient's meals, and for up to 2 hours afterward, monitor him closely for any of the above signs and symptoms. If any appear, notify the doctor.

However, you can help minimize or prevent these signs or symptoms by managing your patient's diet properly. Follow these guidelines when caring for a patient who's had a gastric resection:
• Provide needed liquids 1 hour before or after meals; never during meals. Increased fluid intake during meals will worsen the syndrome's signs and symptoms.
• Place your patient in a low Fowler's position for 30 to 60 minutes after meals. This slows food and fluid movement into the intestine.
• Provide your patient daily with six small, high protein, high fat, low carbohydrate meals. As you know, high protein and fat foods stay in the stomach longer, delaying movement to the intestine.
• Administer anticholinergic drugs to decrease GI activity, and antispasmodic drugs to slow food passage into the intestine, as ordered.

In addition, encourage your patient to plan and maintain a proper diet. Emphasize the importance of controlling or preventing dumping syndrome's signs and symptoms.

*Available in both the United States and in Canada

Preparing your patient for a gastric resection

If your patient is scheduled for gastric resection, he'll probably be worried how the surgery will affect his lifestyle. Do your best to reassure him in your preop patient teaching sessions. Encourage him to ask questions and answer them honestly, choosing words he can understand. For example, explain:
• why he needs surgery.
• how he'll be cared for after surgery (see pages 76 and 77). Also, describe any tubes (such as nasogastric), I.V. lines, or other equipment that he'll have.
• how the loss of part or all his stomach will affect his diet initially, as well as later.

Instruct him how to turn in bed and to use his diaphragm to cough and deep breathe at least once every hour. Explain that these actions help prevent postop pulmonary and vascular complications such as pneumonia and thrombosis. In addition, teach him how to use an incentive spirometer.

Tell your patient to expect some pain as he breathes or coughs. But, remind him that he'll receive pain medication when he needs it. Show him how to minimize possible abdominal pain by splinting his incision with a pillow. (For details, see the NURSING PHOTOBOOK *Providing Respiratory Care.*)

Remember, your patient may forget much of this preop teaching because he's frightened and worried about the surgery's outcome. So, you'll need to reinforce your teaching after surgery.

The doctor may want him transferred to the intensive care unit (ICU) after surgery. If possible, show him the unit before surgery.

Gastrostomy care

Caring for a patient with a gastric resection

1 *Consider this situation: 40-year-old Albert Schmidt has just returned to your floor after a gastric resection. He has a clamped nasogastric (NG) tube and an I.V. of normal saline solution in place. Do you know how to care for his special needs? If you're unsure, follow these guidelines carefully:*

Begin by reassuring Mr. Schmidt. Explain each procedure to him as you perform it. Then, place him in a low to semi-Fowler's position, whichever is most comfortable. Either position will make it easier for him to breathe and prevent him from aspirating gastric contents if he vomits.

Continue to take Mr. Schmidt's vital signs every 2 hours, or as ordered, until his condition stabilizes. Also, carefully monitor his intake and output and record it on his chart.

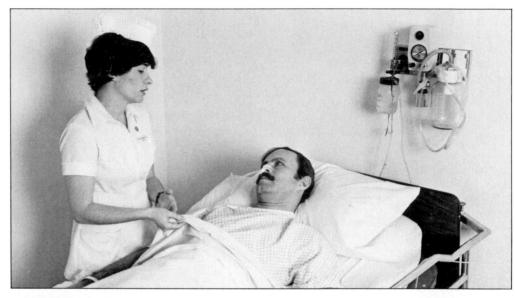

2 Next, unclamp the NG tube and attach it to intermittent low suction, as ordered. Be sure to provide good mouth care while the NG tube's in place.

Important: Never irrigate an NG tube after a gastric resection without a doctor's order. Doing so may tear the patient's sutures.

[Inset] Check the tube's drainage periodically. Record the color, consistency, and amount of the drainage. Remember, for about 12 hours postop, the drainage will appear bloody. However, if after 12 hours the drainage still appears bloody, notify the doctor. Your patient may have bleeding at the internal suture line.

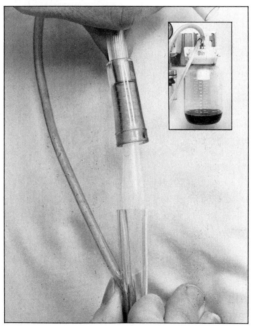

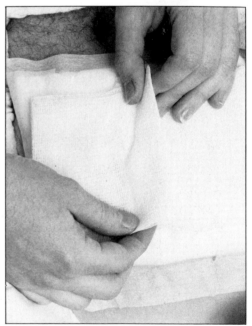

3 Now, inspect your patient's dressing. If you see any drainage, circle it on the dressing, mark the time, and sign your initials. Then, in your nurses' notes, be sure to document the color, consistency, and amount. Continue to check his dressing every 2 to 4 hours, as ordered. Stay alert for increased or bloody drainage. If you see either, notify the doctor.

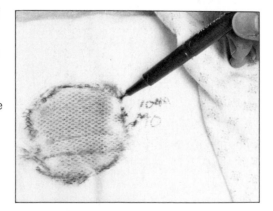

4 About 24 hours postop, the doctor will change Mr. Schmidt's dressing. But suppose the dressing becomes wet or soiled before that time? Reinforce the dressing with 4"x4" sterile gauze pads, as shown. Tape the pads in place.

After the doctor changes the first dressing, you'll change subsequent dressings daily, or whenever soiled, as ordered. When you do, use strict aseptic technique.

5 Has the doctor inserted a Penrose drain at or near your patient's incision site? If so, observe the amount and type of drainage and record this in your notes.

Immediately after surgery, the drainage will be pinkish. After 48 hours, it should be yellowish. But if the drainage is dark red (indicating internal bleeding), purulent (indicating infection), or bile-colored (indicating a suture line separation at the duodenal stump), notify the doctor. He may want you to prepare Mr. Schmidt for surgery.

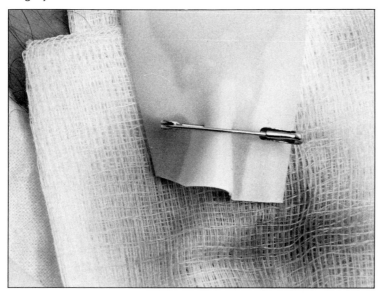

6 To keep the dressing clean, protect your patient's skin, re-duce the need for frequent dress-ing changes, and to allow for more accurate drainage records, apply skin barrier and an ostomy pouch over your patient's Penrose drain.

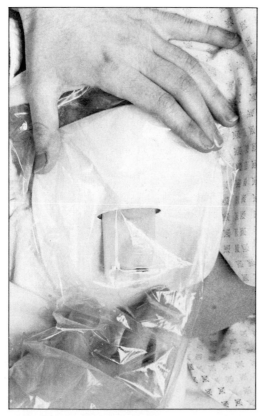

7 To prevent venous stasis and thrombophlebitis, put antiembo-lism stockings on your patient, as shown here. For more details, see the NURSING PHOTOBOOK *Caring for Surgical Patients*. In addition, make sure the patient ambulates early—usually the first day postop—as ordered.

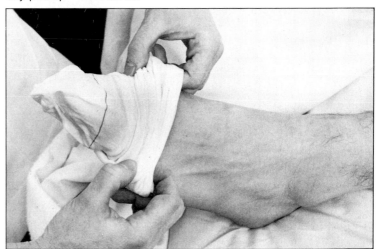

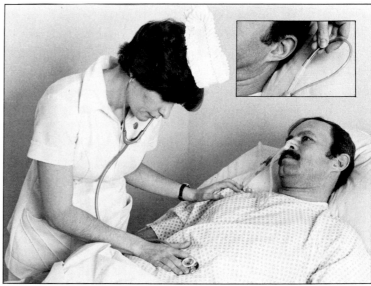

8 As you auscultate your patient's abdomen daily, listen for the return of his bowel sounds. After they return, the doctor may instruct you to clamp Mr. Schmidt's NG tube on a specific schedule. Doing so helps determine how tolerant your patient will be to NG tube removal.

If your patient complains of nausea or begins vomiting when the tube's clamped, unclamp it immediately and attach the tube to suction. Record the amount, color, and consistency of the vomitus, and notify the doctor.

But if everything's okay, the doctor will order your patient's tube clamped continuously (see inset). In that case, give Mr. Schmidt small amounts of clear liquids, as ordered. If he tolerates the liquids, remove the tube and gradually increase his diet, as ordered. Also, look for signs and symptoms of dumping syndrome (see page 75 for details). If you see any, notify the doctor.

Finally, document all procedures in your notes.

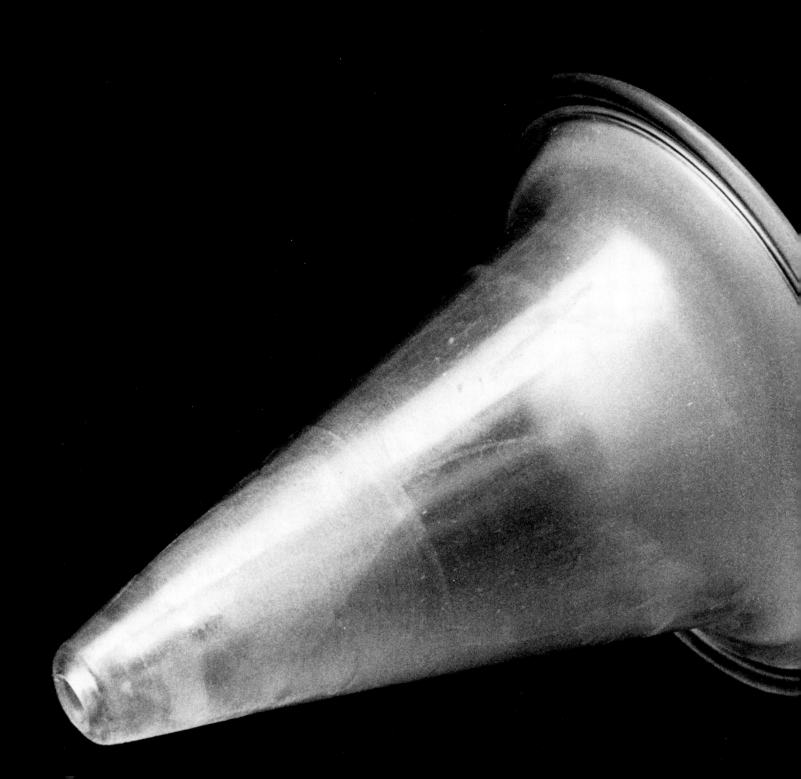

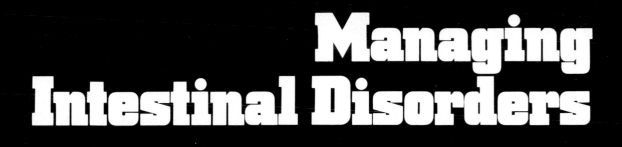

Managing Intestinal Disorders

Stoma care
Intestinal tube care
Special problems

Stoma care

Let's imagine you're caring for a patient with a new colostomy. The doctor orders an irrigation. Do you know how to do it? Do you know how to apply a reusable pouch using the one-piece method? Or how to teach your patient to clean his reusable pouch?

What if your patient has a continent ileostomy? Do you know how to properly pass the catheter through the nipple valve? What to do if the drainage is too thick?

Do you really know all you should about ostomies? For example, do you know why the doctor would perform a transverse colostomy? How to help prepare your patient for ostomy surgery? What to do if your patient's faceplate doesn't adhere properly to his skin?

Read this section for the answers to these questions. We've included valuable nursing tips, home care aids, and charts to familiarize you with ostomy equipment and locations.

Diseases and disorders requiring ostomies: Nurses' guide

How much do you know about the diseases and disorders requiring ostomies? This chart can familiarize you with the most common ones. It indicates their signs and symptoms, and also explains how a doctor may diagnose the problem.

Crohn's disease (regional ileitis)

Signs and symptoms
- Mild diarrhea four to six times daily, usually without blood. Can alternate with constipation.
- Chronic, steady ache in right lower abdominal quadrant, mimicking appendicitis when pain's acute
- Abdominal cramps relieved by bowel movement
- Chronic fever, usually no higher than 102° F. (38.9° C.)
- Possible intestinal abscesses or fistulas
- Anorexia and weight loss
- Family history of disease
- Recurring periods of exacerbation and remission of symptoms

Diagnostic indicators
- Small bowel series
- Stool exam to rule out bacterial or viral dysentery
- Lower GI endoscopy (with biopsy), to differentiate from ulcerative colitis
- Barium enema to confirm diagnosis

Intervention
- Limit diarrhea-causing foods.
- Administer steroid drugs in acute stages, as ordered by the doctor. Steroid drugs may increase the possibility of patient developing anal and abdominal fistulas and can prevent healing.
- Administer codeine or Lomotil*, as ordered, to control diarrhea.
- Prepare patient for surgery, if ordered. Doctor may perform colon-to-colon, or ileum-to-colon resection (60% recurrence rate), or a total colectomy with ileostomy (25% recurrence rate). Condition usually treated medically for as long as possible.

*Available in both the United States and in Canada

Diverticulitis

Signs and symptoms
- Aching pain and tenderness in left lower abdominal quadrant
- Referred suprapubic pain
- Low-grade fever
- Nausea, vomiting, and anorexia
- Leukocytosis
- Pencil-shaped stools
- Constipation. In rare cases, diarrhea
- Sudden massive intestinal hemorrhage

Diagnostic indicators
- Barium enema
- Lower GI endoscopy (with biopsy) to rule out colorectal cancer

Intervention
- Discontinue oral feeding, as ordered, to rest bowel.
- Administer I.V. fluids, as ordered.
- Be prepared to administer total parenteral nutrition (TPN), as ordered.
- Administer stool softeners or dietary bulk, as ordered.
- Be prepared to administer antibiotics and pain medication, as ordered.
- If the patient's bowel is perforated or obstructed, prepare him for a temporary diverting colostomy, or bowel resection, as ordered by the doctor.
- Provide patient with complete bed rest.

Colorectal cancer

Signs and symptoms
Right colon
- Vague, dull, uncharacteristic abdominal pain
- Dark red blood in stool
- Anemia
- Mass in right lower quadrant
- Weight loss
Left colon
- Gas pains and cramps
- Bright red blood mixed in stool
- Pencil-shaped stools
- Patient has increased his use of laxatives or enemas.
- Acute, large, bowel obstruction causing progressive abdominal distention, pain, vomiting, and constipation.
- Onset may be insidious.
- Weight loss
Rectum
- Bright red blood coating stool
- Pain (in advanced stage)
- Spasmodic contraction of anal sphincter with pain and persistent urge to empty bowel
- Pencil-shaped stools
- Weight loss (late sign)

Diagnostic indicators
- Digital rectal exam
- Barium enema
- Serum-hemoglobin level to determine anemia
- Endoscopy with biopsy
- Stool exam to determine presence of occult blood

Intervention
- Get ready to administer total parenteral nutrition (TPN), as ordered.
- Prepare patient for surgery, if ordered. Doctor may remove tumor and perform an end-to-end anastomosis, or a partial or total colectomy with colostomy or ileostomy.
- Be prepared to administer blood transfusions, as ordered.
- If patient has advanced cancer, keep him as comfortable as possible. Give him medication for pain, as ordered.
- Administer chemotherapy, as ordered. Observe for side effects, such as nausea, vomiting, and alopecia.

Ulcerative colitis

Signs and symptoms
- Weakness with a general feeling of illness
- Frequent, bloody diarrhea that's initially mild, then more severe, and finally fulminating.
- Extreme abdominal tenderness with muscle guarding, which may indicate peritonitis caused by a perforated bowel
- Fever: 100° to 102° F. (37.8° to 38.9° C.)
- Abdominal cramps
- Malnutrition and dehydration; anorexia
- Anemia with leukocytosis

Diagnostic indicators
- Lower GI endoscopy (with biopsy)
- Complete blood count (CBC)
- Barium enema
- Stool exam to rule out parasites

Intervention
- Restrict patient's intake of milk, fruit, and vegetables, as ordered.
- Administer Lomotil* for diarrhea and prednisone to help reduce inflammation, as ordered by the doctor.
- Provide bed rest for patient
- In severe cases, make sure patient follows a milk-free diet with restricted fiber intake, as ordered. Also administer corticotropin (ACTH) by I.V., as ordered.
- In fulminant cases, follow for 10 days the guidelines listed above, as ordered. If patient doesn't respond satisfactorily, or if biopsy indicates cancerous or precancerous cells, the doctor will perform total colectomy with an ileostomy to treat condition. Without surgery, death may result.

Stoma care

Nurses' guide to ostomies

How familiar are you with ostomies? For example, can you differentiate a descending from a transverse colostomy? If your patient has a loop ileostomy, do you know where to check for mucous drainage?

The chart on these pages answers these questions and gives you specific information on different types of ostomies. In addition, follow these general guidelines when caring for a patient with any type of ostomy:

• Empty your patient's ostomy pouch when it's one third to one half full. If the fluid level gets too high, the seal will come loose.
• Check for stoma leakage. If you see any, change the pouch immediately. The drainage can irritate the skin around the stoma.
• When changing an ostomy pouch, wash the area around the stoma with warm tap water, and mild, nonperfumed soap.
• Apply a skin barrier to the area around the stoma, to protect the skin from irritation.
• Control drainage odor with an odor-proof pouch and pouch deodorant. Use internal deodorants (for example, bismuth subgallate) only as ordered by the doctor.
• Recommend the use of a pouch cover. It will increase your patient's comfort by reducing perspiration trapped between his skin and the ostomy pouch. It will also make the pouch more aesthetically pleasing during sexual intimacy.

Ascending colostomy (Middle or upper right side of abdomen)

Reason for surgery
• Perforating sigmoid diverticulitis
• Hirschsprung's disease
• Rectovaginal fistula
• Penetrating trauma
• Bowel obstruction from inoperable tumor in colon

Drainage
• Watery or semisolid, usually constant
• Foul-smelling

Nursing considerations
• Fit patient with odor-proof, drainable pouch.
• Do not irrigate stoma.

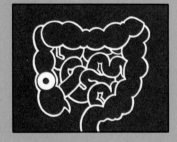

Transverse colostomy (Upper abdomen, near midline)

Reason for surgery
• Same as for ascending colostomy (described above)

Drainage
• Semiliquid or very soft
• Foul-smelling

Nursing considerations
• Fit patient with an odor-proof, drainable pouch.
• Do not irrigate stoma, unless ordered by doctor.
• If your patient has a double-barreled colostomy or loop colostomy, check for mucous discharge at the distal (inactive) opening. Fecal matter will drain from the proximal (active) opening. Tell patient to expect occasional rectal drainage.

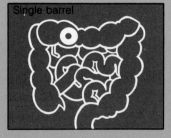

Single barrel

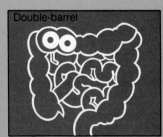

Double-barrel

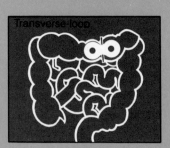

Transverse-loop

Intestinal tract

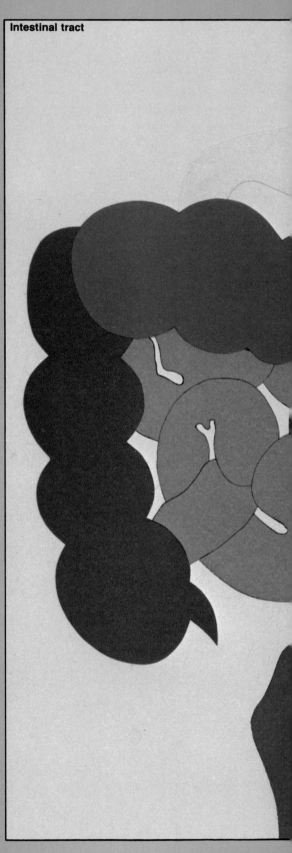

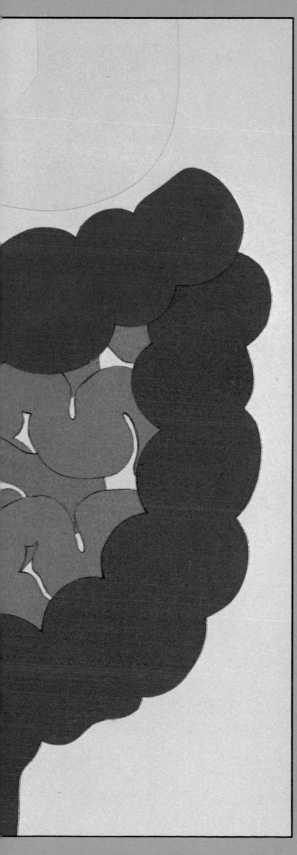

Ileostomy   (Lower right abdominal quadrant)

Reason for surgery
- Ulcerative colitis
- Crohn's disease
- Familial polyposis

Drainage
- Liquid or pastelike, constant
- Foul-smelling

Nursing considerations
- Make sure patient has odor-proof, drainable pouch.
- If your patient has a loop ileostomy, check for mucous drainage from distal (inactive) opening. Fecal material will drain from proximal (active) opening.

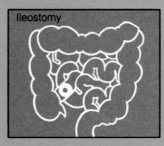

Ileostomy

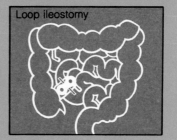

Loop ileostomy

Sigmoid colostomy   (Lower left abdominal quadrant)

Reason for surgery
- Cancer of rectum
- Cancer of sigmoid colon
- Chronic diverticulitis

Drainage
- Soft to firm; resembles normal bowel movement. May be semiliquid after surgery.

Nursing considerations
- Immediately after surgery, attach drainable pouch. After the colostomy's regulated, your patient may choose to use a closed pouch or a stoma cap. But if diarrhea develops, he may want to use a drainable pouch.
- Teach your patient how to regulate his colostomy through diet.
- Irrigate colostomy, only as ordered by the doctor or enterostomal therapist.

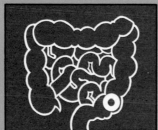

Continent ileostomy   (Lower right abdominal quadrant)

Reason for surgery
- Ulcerative colitis
- Familial polyposis

Drainage
- Liquid or pastelike
- Foul-smelling

Nursing considerations
- Patients with this type of ostomy usually do not need to wear any pouch. Intermittent catheterization normally controls drainage and gas.
- After surgery, be prepared to catheterize patient's stoma so drainage flows continuously into a drainage bag, as ordered by the doctor.
- If patient has mucous discharge, recommend use of a small, closed pouch. Or, place a small, absorbent dressing over stoma.
- Use a No. 28 Silastic catheter to remove drainage from pouch.
- Advise patient that pouch capacity will increase to 750 to 1,000 ml within 6 months. Catheterization frequency will decrease to every 5 to 6 hours.
- If drainage is very thick, instill 30 to 40 ml of warm tap water into pouch before catheterization, as ordered by doctor.
- Immediately after catheterization, use warm tap water to clean stoma thoroughly.
- Instruct patient to avoid eating fibrous foods; for example, popcorn and nuts. These foods may obstruct nipple valve or catheter. Remind patient to chew food thoroughly.

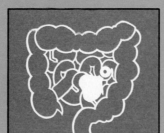

Stoma care

Preparing your patient for an ostomy

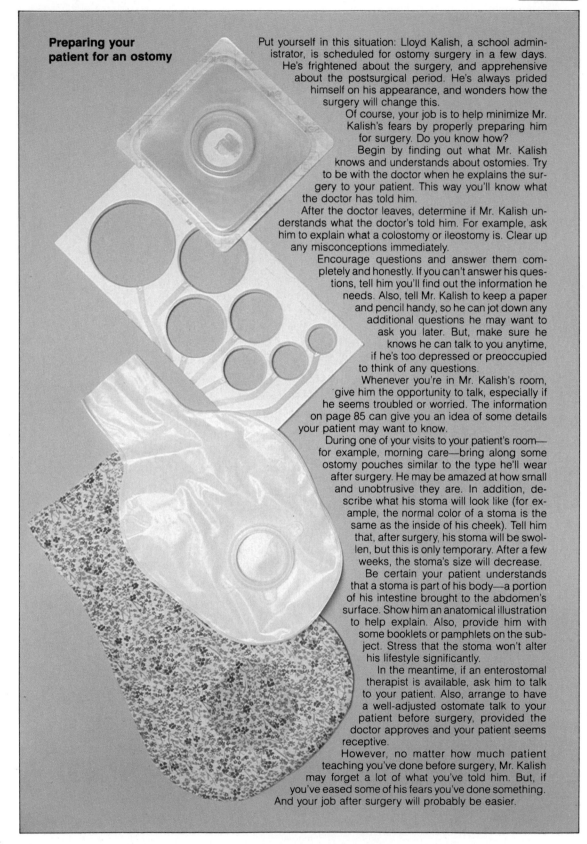

Put yourself in this situation: Lloyd Kalish, a school administrator, is scheduled for ostomy surgery in a few days. He's frightened about the surgery, and apprehensive about the postsurgical period. He's always prided himself on his appearance, and wonders how the surgery will change this.

Of course, your job is to help minimize Mr. Kalish's fears by properly preparing him for surgery. Do you know how?

Begin by finding out what Mr. Kalish knows and understands about ostomies. Try to be with the doctor when he explains the surgery to your patient. This way you'll know what the doctor has told him.

After the doctor leaves, determine if Mr. Kalish understands what the doctor's told him. For example, ask him to explain what a colostomy or ileostomy is. Clear up any misconceptions immediately.

Encourage questions and answer them completely and honestly. If you can't answer his questions, tell him you'll find out the information he needs. Also, tell Mr. Kalish to keep a paper and pencil handy, so he can jot down any additional questions he may want to ask you later. But, make sure he knows he can talk to you anytime, if he's too depressed or preoccupied to think of any questions.

Whenever you're in Mr. Kalish's room, give him the opportunity to talk, especially if he seems troubled or worried. The information on page 85 can give you an idea of some details your patient may want to know.

During one of your visits to your patient's room—for example, morning care—bring along some ostomy pouches similar to the type he'll wear after surgery. He may be amazed at how small and unobtrusive they are. In addition, describe what his stoma will look like (for example, the normal color of a stoma is the same as the inside of his cheek). Tell him that, after surgery, his stoma will be swollen, but this is only temporary. After a few weeks, the stoma's size will decrease.

Be certain your patient understands that a stoma is part of his body—a portion of his intestine brought to the abdomen's surface. Show him an anatomical illustration to help explain. Also, provide him with some booklets or pamphlets on the subject. Stress that the stoma won't alter his lifestyle significantly.

In the meantime, if an enterostomal therapist is available, ask him to talk to your patient. Also, arrange to have a well-adjusted ostomate talk to your patient before surgery, provided the doctor approves and your patient seems receptive.

However, no matter how much patient teaching you've done before surgery, Mr. Kalish may forget a lot of what you've told him. But, if you've eased some of his fears you've done something. And your job after surgery will probably be easier.

Helping your patient understand his ostomy

Chances are, a patient with an ostomy will have apprehensions about his lifestyle after surgery. Encourage him to ask questions, and answer them honestly. Remember, to your patient, an ostomy may seem more devastating than it actually is. But, if you help him understand his ostomy and its care, you may be able to alleviate some of his stress. Here are some answers to questions your patient may ask:

Patient's question:
Will I have an odor?
How to answer:
If your patient cleans his reusable pouch or changes his disposable pouch on a regular schedule, he probably won't have odor problems. But, for additional security, suggest a pouch deodorant. Be sure to remind your patient to notify his doctor if he develops an extremely foul stool odor. He may have an infection, although the odor may be diet related.

Patient's question:
Will I have to change the way I dress?
How to answer:
Reassure your patient that he'll be able to wear his regular clothes, as long as belts do not lie directly over his stoma. Ostomy pouches are undetectable, even under swimsuits, because they're made to lie flat against the body.

But, if your female patient asks about wearing a girdle, recommend that she wear a lightweight, stretch type. A heavy, tight girdle may injure her stoma, or may cause drainage to pool around it, which could loosen the adhesive seal.

Patient's question:
Can I participate in sports?
How to answer:
Usually, a patient with an ostomy can participate in most sports. Tell your patient to check with his doctor. The doctor may want him to avoid rough contact sports, such as wrestling, ice hockey, and football. He may also restrict your patient from participating in some individual sports; for example, weight lifting and shot putting. As you probably know, those sports strain abdominal wall muscles, and may cause a hernia in the stomal area.

Remind your patient that swimming is a sport he'll probably be able to participate in. If he plans to swim, warn him to eat lightly, empty his pouch, and seal it securely before entering the water.

In addition, suggest he wear a pouch support—for example, a wide-belted athletic supporter— under his swimsuit. Your female patient may want to wear the type of girdle sold for swimwear.

Patient's question:
Should I wear my pouch when taking a bath or shower?
How to answer:
In most cases, doing so is a matter of preference. Soap and water will not hurt a patient's stoma, as long as the shower stream is not hitting it full force. If your patient feels uncomfortable about stoma drainage leaking into the bath or shower, he may want to wear his pouch. If he does, tell him to make sure the adhesive seal is watertight. He can ensure this by applying extra tape around the edge of the pouch opening.

Patient's question:
Must I eat a special diet?
How to answer:
Explain to your patient that his doctor may put him on a low-residue diet for the first few weeks after surgery. This will give his bowel a rest. Inform him when he can return to his regular diet.

If your patient was on a special diet before surgery (such as one for diabetes), tell him he'll return to it after surgery. Also, remind him that foods that cause digestive problems before surgery will probably continue to do so after surgery. Stress the importance of chewing food thoroughly. In addition, suggest he limit his intake of hard-to-digest foods, such as whole corn, nuts, and sunflower seeds. Review with your patient the foods which may cause foul-smelling gas; for example, onions, eggs, cabbage, beer, and certain cheeses. Advise your patient to consume smaller portions of these foods, or to avoid them entirely.

Patient's question:
Can I travel?
How to answer:
With advance preparation, your patient will be able to travel wherever and whenever he wants. However, recommend he always keep his ostomy equipment with him, because luggage checked through to his destination may get lost. Also, remind him to take along enough ostomy supplies for the entire trip, if possible If your patient wears a reusable pouch, he may want to pack some disposable pouches as a precaution. Instruct him to find out in advance where he can buy supplies he may need as he travels.

Before any long trip, tell your patient to check with his doctor. The doctor may want to prescribe medication for diarrhea or constipation, if either should develop.

If your patient plans a trip to a foreign country, suggest he buy or borrow an up-to-date directory of English-speaking doctors. If he needs additional help planning the medical considerations of his trip, suggest he contact his local ostomy chapter.

In addition, warn him to use only potable water for irrigations.

Patient's question:
Is it possible and safe for me to have a baby?
How to answer:
A woman with an ostomy can become pregnant and have a normal pregnancy. However, she should discuss the subject with her doctor before she becomes pregnant. In some cases, the doctor may recommend that a patient wait a year or so after ostomy surgery before becoming pregnant. This allows her body to recover completely.

Patient's question:
How will my ostomy affect my sex life?
How to answer:
If your patient had a satisfying sex life before surgery, it will usually remain so after surgery. Emphasize that the stoma can't be injured by close physical contact. And, the ostomy pouch, if applied correctly, will cause no problems. You may want to recommend that your patient empty the pouch before sexual intercourse. He or she may also want to use a pouch cover.

If your female patient's had surgery in the perineal area, she may experience some discomfort during intercourse until the wound heals.

Rarely will a female patient have a physical sexual dysfunction from the ostomy. But, a male patient may experience temporary impotence. Others, who have had an ostomy because of bladder or rectal cancer, may have permanent nerve damage. In this case, encourage your patient and his partner to experiment sexually to attain satisfactory relations.

Occasionally, though, a patient's sexual dysfunction may be psychological. In this situation, encourage the patient to see his doctor to rule out any physical complications. Then, if your patient and his partner still have difficulties adjusting sexually, suggest they see a professional counselor.

Patient's question:
Can I return to work?
How to answer:
If your patient has an occupation that requires heavy, physical labor—for example, a construction worker or meat packer —he may not be able to resume it exactly as before. Under most circumstances, however, he can return to his job as soon as he regains his strength and the doctor says it's okay.

Patient's question:
How do I know if my equipment is working correctly?
How to answer:
A properly fitted ostomy pouch will stay secured to your patient's body and won't interfere with vigorous activity. You or an enterostomal therapist (if your hospital has one on staff) should help him choose the pouch best suited to his needs.

Patient's question:
What can I do about gas filling up my pouch?
How to answer:
For starters, advise your patient to avoid foods that cause gas. Also, tell him to try using a disposable or reusable pouch with a gas filter. By gently pressing on the pouch, he can force the gas out through the filter. For a drainable pouch without a gas filter, tell your patient to open the clip at the bottom of the pouch and drain the contents. This allows the gas to escape.

Remember: Before your patient leaves the hospital, give him the name, address, and telephone number of his local ostomy association. They'll be able to answer any additional questions, and provide continued emotional support.

Stoma care

Choosing ostomy equipment

If your patient has a colostomy or ileostomy, you'll want to help him choose the ostomy equipment that best suits his needs. When recommending a product, always consider your patient's comfort and capabilities. But, also give some thought to his finances.

On the following pages, we'll show you several different types of ostomy pouches. Study this information carefully.

Disposable drainable pouch with attached skin barrier

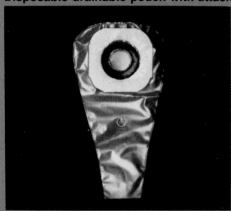 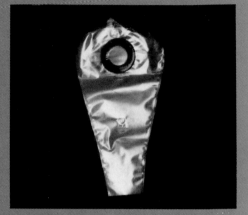

Hollister karaya seal drainable stoma pouch Transparent or opaque, odor-proof plastic pouch with pre-attached karaya seal. Fits stoma openings from 1" to 3" (2.5 to 7.6 cm). Some models may have microporous adhesive or belt tabs. The pouch at left features a karaya seal with microporous adhesives. The pouch at right has a karaya seal with belt tabs.
Indication For patient who needs to empty pouch frequently; for example, a patient with a new colostomy or ileostomy, or a patient with diarrhea. Bottom opening allows easy drainage of contents. May be used permanently or temporarily, replacing it with a reusable pouch when stoma size stabilizes. Especially useful for one-step attachment when skin barrier is used.

Two-piece reusable pouch

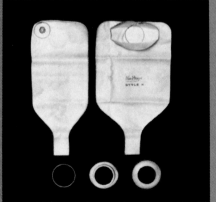

Nu-hope ileostomy pouch Nonallergenic, white plastic drainable pouch with separate custom-made faceplate and O-ring. Some pouches have pressure valve for gas release. With repeated use, has 4 to 6 month life span.
Indications Primarily for the patient who always uses a pouch with his ileostomy.

Stoma cap

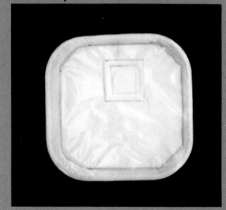

Hollister stoma cap Lightweight plastic square with attached adhesive and absorbent pad with charcoal deodorizing filter.
Indications For patient with regulated colostomy. This product controls odors and absorbs mucous secretions.

Irrigator drain

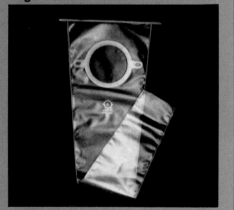

Hollister combination cone tube Clear plastic disposable drain with top opening for cone or colon tube insertion, and long sleeve for drainage into toilet. Top closure strip prevents splashing. Fits stoma openings from 2" to 3" (5.1 to 7.6 cm).
Indications For a colostomy patient who uses irrigation to regulate his bowel functions. Although it's disposable, drain can be used several times.

Disposable closed-end pouch

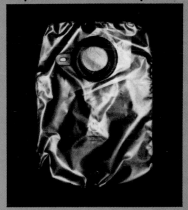 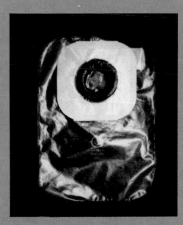 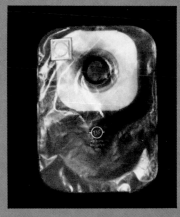 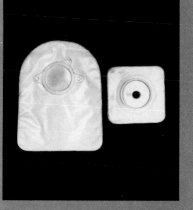

Hollister stoma pouch Clear, odor-proof plastic. Available with adhesive seal, belt tab, skin barrier, and carbon filter for gas release. Fits stoma openings from 1" to 3" (2.5 to 7.6 cm). The pouch at far left features a karaya seal with belt tabs; the middle pouch has karaya and adhesive seals; the pouch at far right has karaya and adhesive seals with a carbon filter.

Indication For a patient with a regulated colostomy. All four pouches shown in this box control odor and are easy-to-use. When patient regulates colostomy, provides additional security and confidence, especially when he's adding new foods to his diet.

Squibb Sur-fit pouch Clear, odor-proof plastic pouch with belt tabs. Snaps to Stomahesive with flange. Fits stoma openings from 1½" to 2¾" (3.8 to 7 cm).

Disposable drainable pouch (with adhesive)

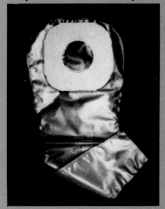 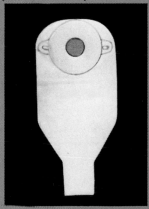 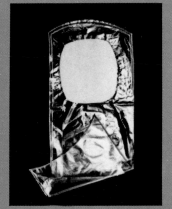

Hollister drainable pouch Clear, odor-proof plastic pouch with pre-attached adhesive square. Fits stoma openings from 1" to 3" (2.5 to 7.6 cm). Some models have belt tabs.

Indication For patient who needs to empty pouch frequently, for example, a patient with a new colostomy or ileostomy, or a patient with diarrhea. Bottom opening allows easy drainage of contents. May be used permanently or temporarily, replacing it with a reusable pouch when stoma size stabilizes.

Nu-hope postop pouch Opaque, odor-proof plastic pouch with belt tabs. Fits stoma openings from ½" to 3" (1.3 to 7.6 cm). Some models have preattached adhesive foam pad.

Bongort® pouch Odor-proof, transparent plastic pouch with adhesive square. Measure and cut adhesive square to fit stoma opening. Especially useful for irregularly shaped stoma.

Disposable drainable pouch

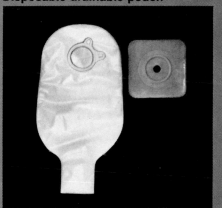

Squibb® Sur-fit® pouch Transparent or opaque, odor-proof pouch with belt tabs. Snaps to Stomahesive® with Sur-fit flange. Fits stoma openings from ½" to 2¾" (1.3 to 7 cm).

Indication Same as for drainable disposable pouch (with adhesive). This product can be removed and replaced without disturbing skin seal.

Stoma care

How to use skin barriers

Various types of skin barriers are available, and choosing what's best for your patient isn't always easy. But, as a rule, consider product availability, cost, patient preference, and skin condition when making your selection.

After you choose the best product for your patient, learn how to apply it properly so you can teach your patient. The following information will familiarize you with various types of skin barriers and the procedures for application.

But, before you apply any barrier, prepare as follows:

Gather the necessary equipment: ostomy pouch, stoma measuring card, adhesive, skin barrier, and scissors. Then, explain the procedure to your patient.

Next, measure the size of your patient's stoma, using a measuring card. For some skin barriers, you'll need this measurement to determine the correct size seal.

Important: Never cut a Reliaseal®, Colly-Seel®, Stomahesive®, or double-faced adhesive foam pad so that the opening's smaller than your patient's stomal measurement. These skin barriers don't stretch and may injure your patient's stoma if they're too small.

Remove your patient's used pouch. Place toilet tissue or a gauze pad over the stoma to absorb any leakage.

🖎 *Nursing tip:* A regular-size tampon held over your patient's stoma will act as a wick, absorbing leakage.

Gently wash the stomal area with warm water to remove the skin barrier and adhesive. Allow the skin to air-dry. Be sure to change the gauze over the stoma, as needed, to keep your patient's skin free of leakage.

The following information will familiarize you with seven types of skin barriers. Read it carefully.

Applying a Colly-Seel ring

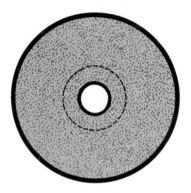

1 Are you using a Colly-Seel ring to protect your patient's skin? If so, cut an opening slightly larger than your patient's stomal measurement.

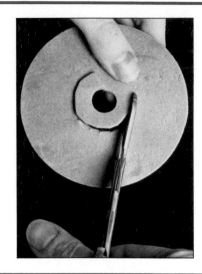

How to use Skin-Prep

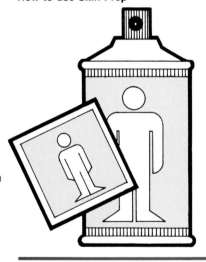

1 Unlike other skin barriers, Skin-Prep™ is a liquid, and requires no measuring or cutting. Instead, you'll brush, wipe, or spray Skin-Prep directly onto the area around your patient's stoma. Here's how to apply Skin-Prep:

First, cover your patient's stoma with a gauze pad. If you're using a brush applicator, carefully apply a thin layer of the plastic coating around the stoma. Let it dry for approximately 30 seconds.

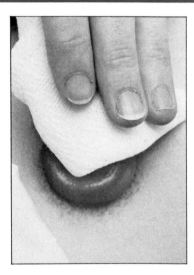

Applying a karaya seal

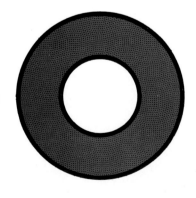

1 As you know, karaya is available as a small ring, giant washer, or sheet. If you have a small ring or giant washer, choose a seal with an opening the same size as your patient's stoma.

Note: Karaya also comes in powder or paste. These can be applied to the skin around the stoma for added protection.

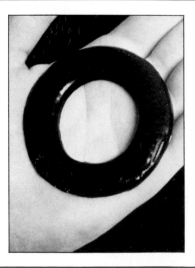

2 Now, moisten the Colly-Seel with warm tap water. Rub water into the ring until it becomes sticky.

Knead the moistened ring to make it more flexible. A flexible ring will fit better around the stoma.

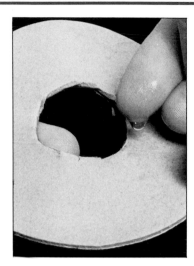

3 Next, center the Colly-Seel over your patient's stoma, as the nurse is doing here. Gently press the ring onto the skin, smoothing out any wrinkles or bubbles.

Now, you're ready to attach the pouch.

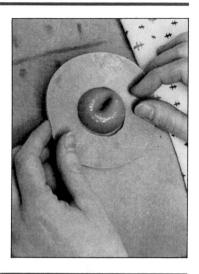

2 Suppose you're using Skin-Prep in individual disposable wipes. To apply, open the package and use the moistened wipe to clean around the stomal area. Make sure the skin's completely covered. Let it dry for 30 seconds.

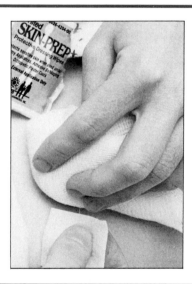

3 Or, if you're using Skin-Prep aerosol, spray around the stomal area evenly. Let it dry for about 30 seconds.

Important: Never spray Skin-Prep directly onto a stoma.

Finally, attach the pouch.

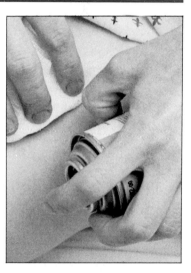

2 Slightly moisten the karaya with a few drops of warm water until it becomes sticky.

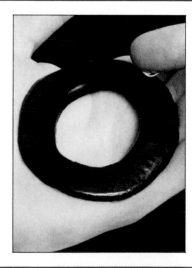

3 Place the seal around your patient's stoma, making sure it fits snugly at the base. Then, gently press the seal, so it adheres to the skin.

Finally, attach the pouch.

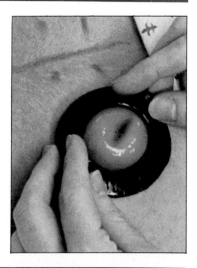

Stoma care

How to use skin barriers continued

Applying Stomahesive

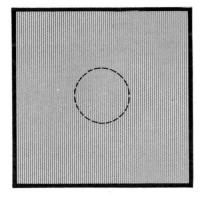

1 To apply Stomahesive, trace your patient's stoma size on the Stomahesive backing.

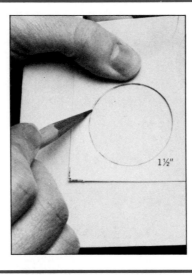

2 Cut out the circle you've traced.
Stomahesive also comes in a powder that can be applied to the skin around the stoma.
Important: Never put Stomahesive on your patient's stoma.

Applying a double-adhesive foam pad

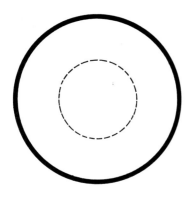

1 Applying a double-adhesive foam pad? If so, try to choose one with an opening the same size as the faceplate (slightly larger than the stoma).
But, if you're using a foam pad without a precut opening, cut an opening the same size as your patient's stoma.

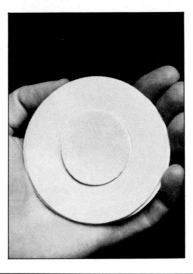

2 Peel the paper backing from one side of the pad. Press the pad's sticky side onto the faceplate.
Note: If you're applying the foam pad to a convex faceplate, you may need to simultaneously remove both pieces of the paper backing to avoid wrinkles.

Applying ReliaSeal

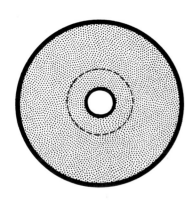

1 If you're applying ReliaSeal skin barrier, cut an opening the same size as the stomal measurement.

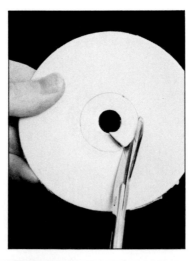

2 Now, remove the white paper covering on the ReliaSeal.

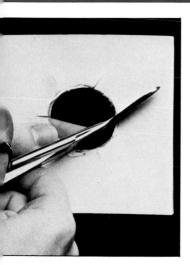

3 Next, remove the Stomahesive backing. Center the sheet, sticky side down, over your patient's stoma. Gently press the sheet on his skin, smoothing out any wrinkles. Hold the Stomahesive in place for 30 seconds.

Now, you're ready to apply the pouch.

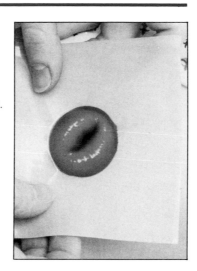

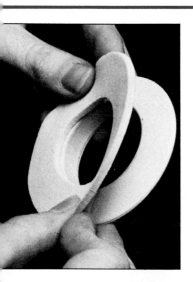

3 Now, peel off the remaining paper backing. Center the faceplate over your patient's stoma and press gently.

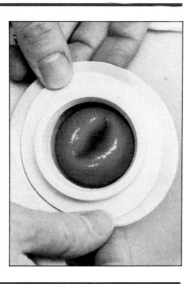

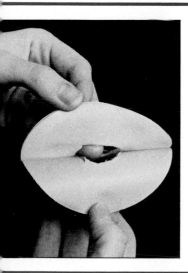

3 Before applying the pouch, peel off the blue paper backing from the ReliaSeal. The adhesive underneath this backing will secure the pouch to the ReliaSeal. Center the ReliaSeal over your patient's stoma, and press gently to remove all wrinkles.

After a few minutes, your patient's body heat will soften the protective gel against his skin. This will secure the seal.

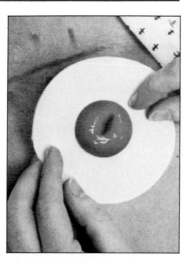

Patch testing your patient's skin

1 *Before applying a new brand of tape, adhesive, or protective gel to the skin around your patient's stoma, patch test his sensitivity to the new product. Here's how:*

First, explain the test procedure to your patient. Then, apply a small patch of the material to be tested to an area that's located away from the stoma and free of excessive hair; for example, his abdomen or his inner arm. In this photostory, we're patch testing skin cement on the patient's arm.

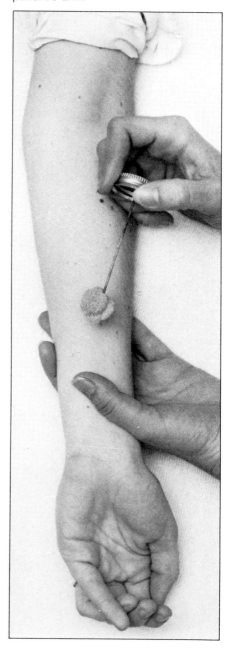

Stoma care

Patch testing your patient's skin continued

2 Now, completely cover the area with nonallergenic tape. Leave the skin cement and tape on his arm for 24 hours, unless he complains of itching or burning, in which case you should remove the tape immediately. Then, wipe the area with cement solvent, and wash it with soap and water. Dry thoroughly. Document in your notes the time and date the cement was applied.

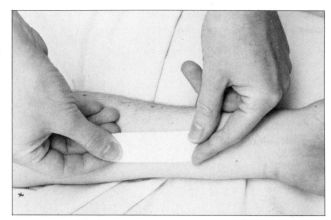

3 After 24 hours, remove the tape and inspect your patient's skin. If everything's okay, your patient probably isn't sensitive to the cement. You'll be able to use the product routinely, although you should continue to check your patient's skin daily for signs of allergic reaction.
Use a gauze pad saturated with cement solvent to wipe the cement from your patient's skin. Clean the area with soap and water, and dry it thoroughly. Document your findings.

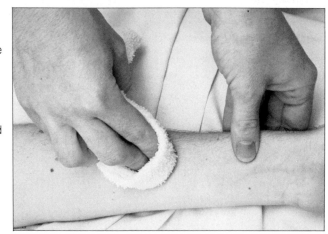

4 What if you note skin redness or your patient complains of burning or itching after you remove the tape? Your patient probably has an allergic reaction.
In this case, wash the patient's skin with soap and water. Dry thoroughly. Choose another type of adhesive and retest the patient's skin, following the same procedure.
[Inset] In some cases, a patient may be allergic only to the tape, and not the cement. If that's so, the redness will occur only in those areas covered by the tape and not the cement.
Finally, remember to document the test results in your nurses' notes.

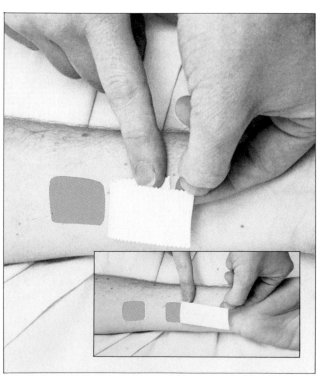

How to apply skin cement

1 *Your patient prefers to use skin cement instead of karaya to attach his pouch to his skin. To apply it properly, follow the instructions below:*
Before applying the cement, check the manufacturer's instructions on the bottle.
Then, apply a small amount of cement to your fingertip or an applicator, as shown here.

2 Use the applicator to evenly apply the cement over the faceplate. Make sure the surface is completely covered, then set aside the faceplate.

3 Now, cover the stoma with a gauze pad to avoid getting cement on the stoma.
Using the applicator, carefully apply a thin layer of cement to your patient's clean, dry skin. Spread the cement evenly around the stoma so it covers an area the same size as the faceplate.

4 Next, following the same procedure, apply another thin coat of cement to the faceplate and to the area around his stoma. Let both surfaces dry until the cement feels tacky.
Finally, attach the faceplate to your patient's skin.

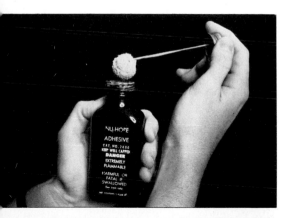

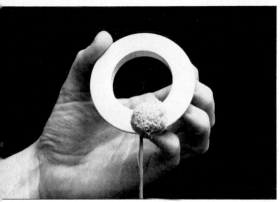

Applying a disposable pouch

1 *Madeline Alby, a 45-year-old dental assistant, has just returned from surgery with a colostomy. The doctor has asked you to apply a disposable ostomy pouch. Do you know how? If you're unsure, follow these steps:*

First, gather the necessary equipment: a drainable, disposable pouch with adhesive square; protective seal (such as Colly-Seel®); pouch closure or rubber band; measuring card; belt or tape; and scissors.

Then, explain the procedure to your patient. Expose the area around her stoma. Drape the other areas of her body to keep her warm and ensure privacy.

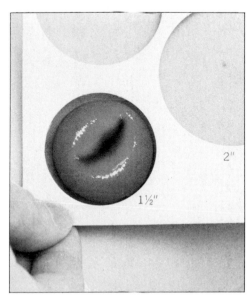

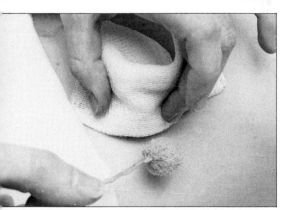

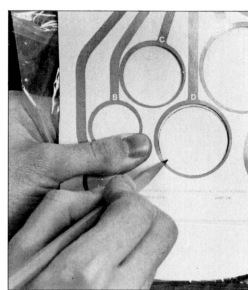

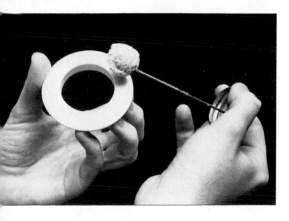

2 Using a measuring card, center one of the larger circles over Ms. Alby's stoma. Continue with smaller circles on the measuring card, until you find the circle that most closely fits her stoma size.

3 Now, with a pencil, trace a circle 1/16" (.2 cm) larger than your patient's stoma onto the pouch's adhesive square.

Important: Immediately after surgery, the stoma will be edematous but will shrink before it reaches a permanent size. You'll need to remeasure your patient's stoma every week—or more often, if indicated—until the edema subsides.

Stoma care

Applying a disposable pouch continued

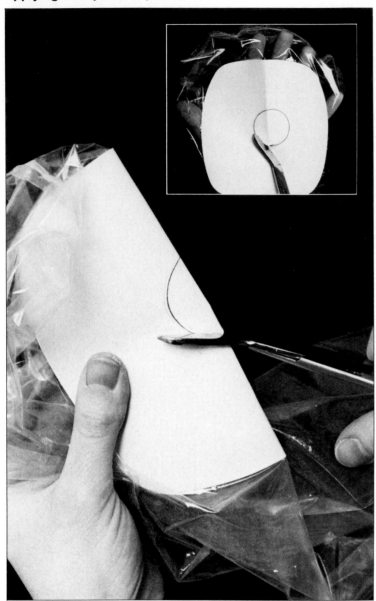

4 Fold the adhesive backing in half, lengthwise. Then cut a half-circle in the adhesive, as shown here. Be sure to keep the pouch away from the adhesive, to prevent cutting through the pouch.

If the pouch has a large opening in the bottom, you can keep the pouch away from the adhesive by slipping your hand up through the pouch and spreading your fingers behind the adhesive, as shown in the inset.

Note: Some disposable pouches have openings precut in standard sizes. If you're applying this type of pouch to your patient, be sure the opening's the proper size.

5 Peel off the backing from the adhesive seal. Then, center the pouch's opening over your patient's stoma. Eliminate any wrinkles. Gently press down, as shown here.

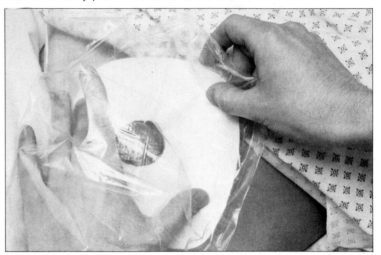

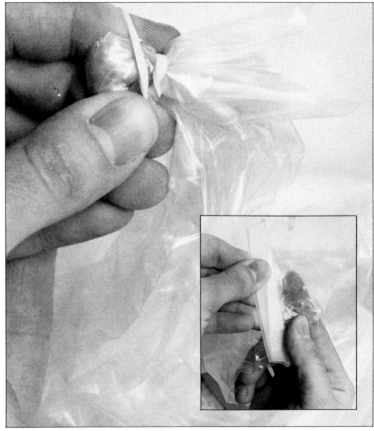

6 Now you're ready to close your patient's pouch. To do this, fanfold the end of the pouch sideways. Turn up the bottom two or three times.

Then, tightly wrap a rubber band around the end of the pouch, as the nurse is doing here. Or, attach a clamp, such as the Hollister drainable pouch clamp, to the bottom (see inset).

Finally, document the entire procedure in your nurses' notes.

How to use a paper guide strip

1 *Caring for a patient with an opaque pouch? If so, you'll want to use a paper guide strip. When attaching your patient's pouch, the guide strip will help you center the faceplate over the stoma.*

First, cut a 6″ (15.2 cm) long strip of a ½″ wide, commercially made paper guide strip.

☙ *Nursing tip:* You can make your own paper guide strip by cutting a strip of inexpensive bond paper ½″ (1.3 cm) wide and 6″ (15.2 cm) long.

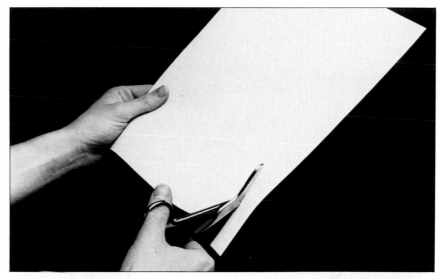

2 Now, shape the strip by wrapping it around your finger, as the nurse is doing in this photo.

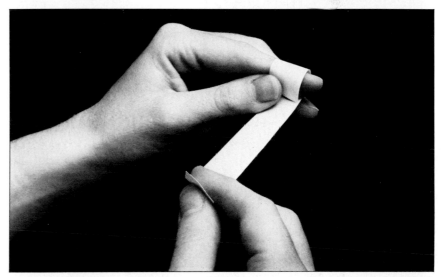

3 Carefully place the strip in the faceplate opening, as shown here. The strip should expand to fit the opening and should protrude slightly.

Finally, center the faceplate over your patient's stoma. Use your fingers to firmly press the adhesive seal to your patient's skin. As you do this, the paper guide will fall into the pouch.

Note: A commercially made paper guide strip will dissolve in the pouch. A handmade strip won't.

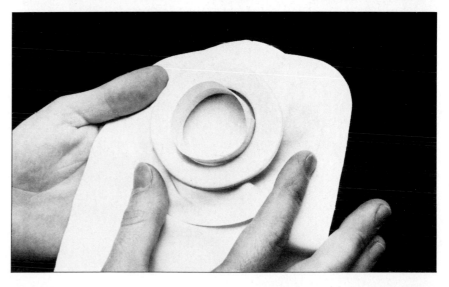

Stoma care

How to apply a reusable pouch: One-piece method

1 *Picture this: During the morning report, you find out that your patient, 65-year-old Tom Mullen, has an ileostomy. Mr. Mullen was admitted to the hospital with organic brain syndrome. When you begin his morning care, you notice the seal of his reusable pouch has loosened. You'll want to apply a clean pouch. Here's how:*

First, gather the following equipment: Nu-hope pouch and faceplate, skin barrier, such as Skin-Prep™, cement or Nu-hope adhesive disc, pouch closure, metal or O-ring, and supporting shield and belt, if desired.

Make sure the patient's room is warm and well lighted. Then, explain the procedure to him, even though he's unconscious. Position him flat on his back with his arms at his sides. Remove the old pouch.

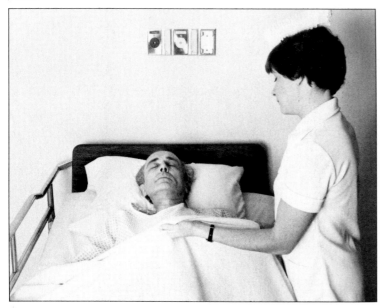

2 Now, lay the pouch on a flat surface, with the cup facing up. Slip the metal ring around the cup. The ring's protruding edge should be against the pouch. Next, fold the cup down over the ring.

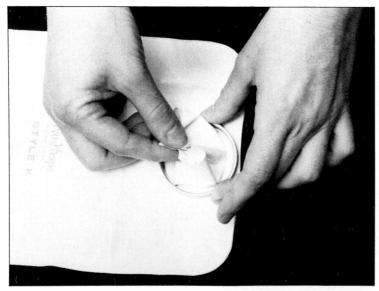

3 Firmly press the faceplate against the ring, and make sure they snap together, to provide a tight seal.

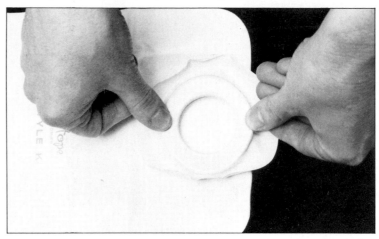

4 Next, place the pouch, faceplate up, on a flat surface. Then, peel off the paper backing from one side of the double-sided adhesive disc.

Then, carefully center the adhesive disc, sticky side down, over the faceplate. Firmly press the disc onto the faceplate.

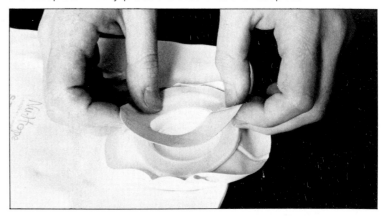

5 Remove the remaining backing from the adhesive disc. Insert a coiled paper guide strip into the faceplate opening.

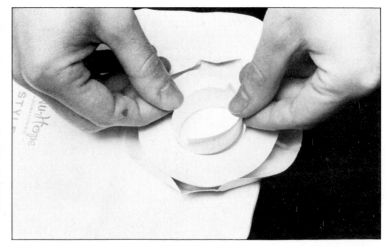

6 Now, clean the area around your patient's stoma with warm water, and dry it thoroughly. Swab the area with a Skin-Prep wipe, which provides waterproof protection. Allow it to dry approximately 30 seconds.

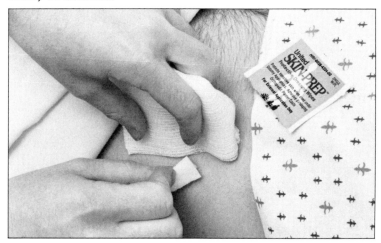

7 Carefully position the assembled pouch over Mr. Mullen's stoma, as the nurse is doing here. The entire surface of the adhesive disc should touch Mr. Mullen's skin. Press firmly against the disc to make sure it's secure. As you do, the paper guide strip will fall into the pouch.

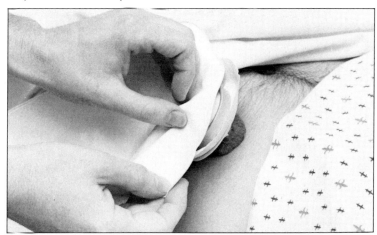

8 Finally, close the bottom of the pouch with a clamp, as shown here.

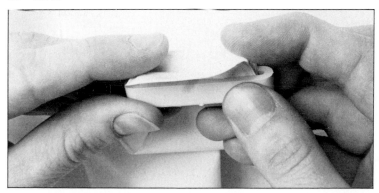

9 Occasionally, you may find that the pouch isn't adequately secured. If it isn't, slip a supporting shield over the pouch and faceplate, making sure it lies flat against Mr. Mullen's skin.

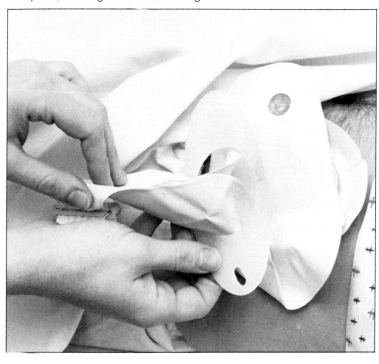

10 Finally, attach a pouch belt to the shield, and secure it around your patient's waist, as shown here. Document the entire procedure in your nurses' notes.

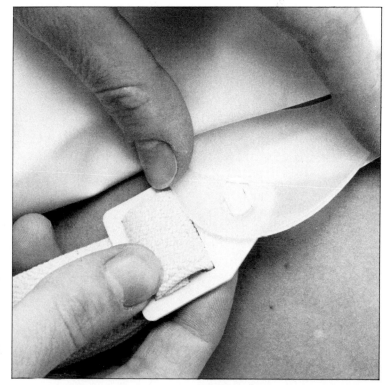

Stoma care

How to apply a reusable pouch: Two-piece method

1 *You may prefer to use the two-piece method to apply Mr. Mullen's reusable pouch. Do you know how to proceed? If you're unsure, follow these steps:*

Begin by gathering the equipment you'll need: a clean pouch and faceplate; skin barrier, such as Skin-Prep™; cement or an adhesive disc; pouch clip or rubber band; metal or rubber O-ring; and a supporting shield and belt, if desired.

Explain the procedure to your patient. Position Mr. Mullen flat in bed with his arms at his sides. Make sure the room's warm and well lighted.

Expose your patient's stoma. Drape the other areas of his body to keep him warm and protect his privacy.

Remove the used pouch.

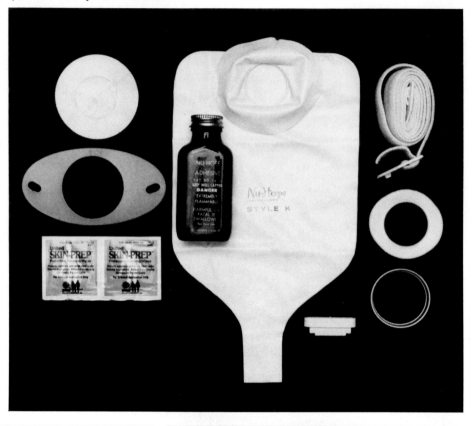

4 Next, clean and dry the skin around your patient's stoma. Wipe the area around the stoma with the moistened Skin-Prep disposable wipe. Allow the site to dry for approximately 30 seconds.

5 Peel the remaining paper backing off the adhesive disc. Center the faceplate over Mr. Mullen's stoma. Gently press around the stoma so the adhesive bonds to his skin. Carefully press out any wrinkles, ensuring a tight seal.

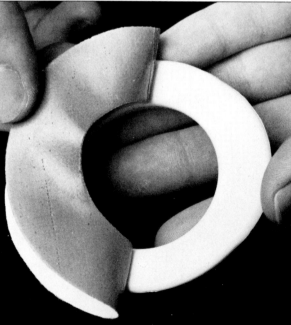

6 Lay the pouch on a flat surface, with the cup facing up. Then, slip the metal ring around the cup. Be sure the ring's protruding edge is against the pouch. Now, fold the cup down over the ring (see inset).

2 Now, measure the size of Mr. Mullen's stoma, as the nurse is doing in this photo. Then, select an adhesive disc with an opening that matches the size of his stoma. Carefully, peel off one side of the disc's paper backing.

3 Center the adhesive disc—sticky side down— over the faceplate. Firmly press the disc over the faceplate, making sure there are no wrinkles or bubbles between the faceplate and the adhesive. Set the faceplate aside.

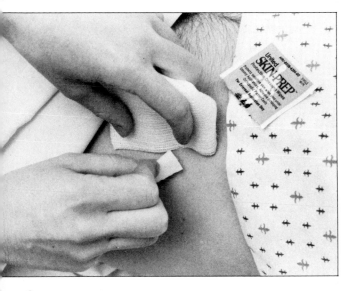

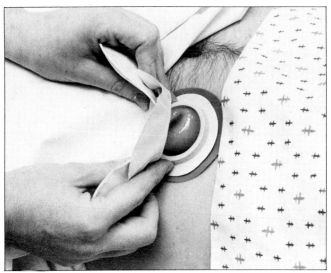

7 To secure the pouch to the faceplate, firmly press the pouch's cup against the faceplate.
  Important: The metal ring should be fully snapped into the faceplate for a tight seal.

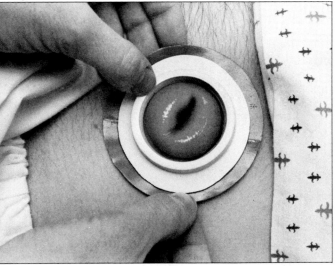

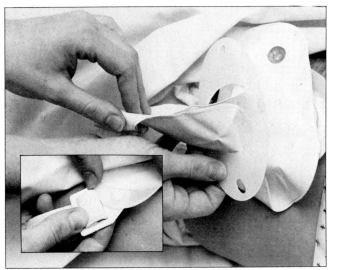

8 If additional support is needed, slip the supporting shield over the pouch and faceplate.
  Then, attach the shield to a belt, as shown in the inset.

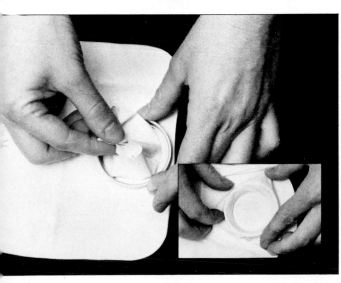

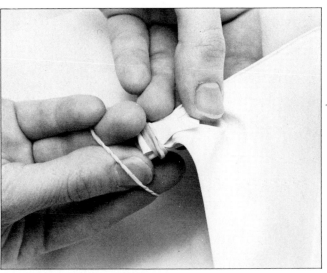

9 Fanfold the end of the pouch sideways. Turn up the bottom two or three times.
  Then, fasten it with a rubber band, as shown here. Or, clamp the bottom of the pouch.
  Document the procedure in your nurses' notes.

Stoma care

How to remove your patient's ostomy pouch

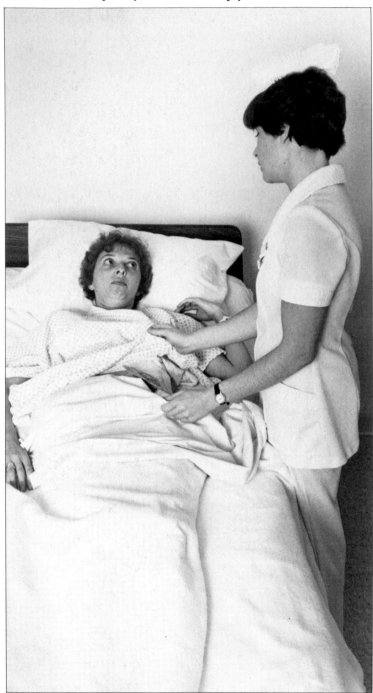

1 *Whenever you change your patient's ostomy pouch, you'll need to first remove her used pouch and clean off the adhesive that remains on her skin.*

To do this, gather the necessary equipment: a clean ostomy pouch; skin barrier, if desired; gauze pads; adhesive solvent; and an eyedropper (if needed).

Note: Some solvents come in presaturated sponges or aerosol sprays.

Explain the procedure to your patient. Then, have her stand up (if possible) or lie flat on her back with her pouch exposed.

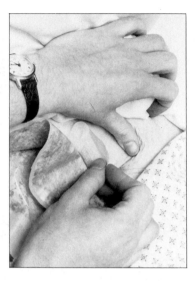

2 Now, hold the skin taut around your patient's stoma, as you gently peel back the top of the adhesive square, as shown here. Then, continue peeling downward.

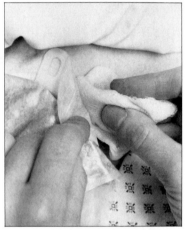

3 Having difficulty removing the pouch? Never use force. Doing so may cause skin abrasion. Instead, try loosening the adhesive.

Here's one way: Wet a gauze pad with warm water. Then, moisten the skin around your patient's faceplate. Slowly peel off the pouch.

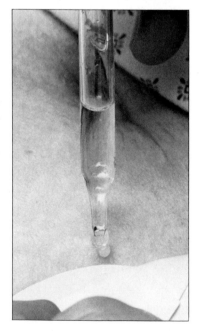

4 However, when skin cement has been used as an adhesive, you may need to use adhesive solvent to loosen it. To do this, fill an eyedropper with solvent. Using the dropper, loosen each edge of the faceplate with a drop or two of solvent. Wait a few seconds, then try to remove the faceplate. If you're unsuccessful, add another drop or two of solvent. Wait a few seconds and try again. Continue this procedure until you remove the faceplate completely.

◤ *Nursing tip:* If you don't have an eyedropper, use a gauze pad moistened with solvent.

Clean and dry the skin around your patient's stoma. Finally, apply a skin barrier (if used) and a new pouch.

Dilating a stoma

1 *Caring for a patient with a new colostomy? If so, the doctor may want you to dilate his stoma before irrigating. Here's how:*

First, assemble the equipment you'll need: an examining glove, gauze pads, and water-soluble lubricant. At this time, also gather the necessary irrigating equipment (see page 102).

Then, explain the procedure to your patient. If the doctor wants him to continue dilating his stoma at home, take this opportunity to teach your patient the dilation procedure.

[Inset] Now, slip the examining glove onto your hand. Squeeze a small amount of lubricant onto your little finger, as shown in this photo.

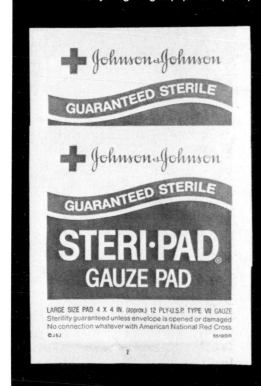
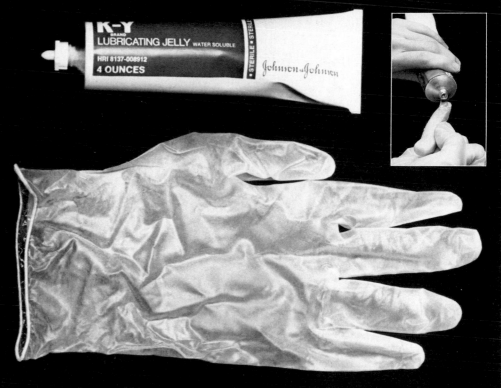
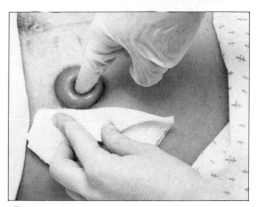

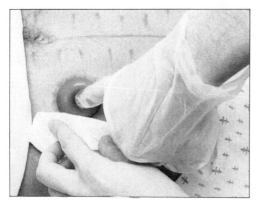

2 Hold several gauze pads under your patient's stoma to protect the skin from stomal drainage. Now, gently, but firmly, insert your little finger 2″ (5 cm) into his stoma. Maintain this position for 1 minute.

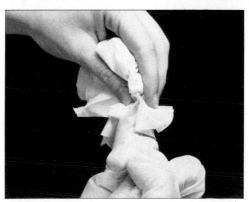

3 Next, remove your finger from your patient's stoma. Wipe your finger with a tissue or gauze pad, as shown here. Remember, a small amount of blood on your finger may be normal if your patient has a new colostomy. However, if you see a large amount of bright red blood, notify the doctor immediately.

4 Now, lubricate your gloved index finger. Insert this finger into your patient's stoma. Maintain this position for 1 minute. Then, remove your finger and wipe it clean.

Finally, lubricate the stoma cone and begin the irrigation procedure. Document the entire procedure in your nurses' notes.

Important: Never dilate a patient's stoma without a doctor's order.

Stoma care

How to irrigate a colostomy

1 *Consider this: Elaine Johnson, a 47-year-old pilot, is a patient in your unit after partial colectomy and formation of a descending colostomy. The doctor has left orders to irrigate Ms. Johnson's colostomy using a colon tube inserted approximately 3" (7.6 cm).*

Do you know how to proceed? If you're unsure, follow these guidelines:

First, prepare for the procedure by gathering the necessary equipment: I.V. pole, bedpan, bed-saver pad, water-soluble lubricant, irrigating set with colon tube or stoma cone tip, stoma irrigator drain, belt, and 1,000 ml warm tap water or irrigating solution, as ordered.

Note: In this photostory, we're using a Hollister® irrigator set with an interchangeable tip.

Then, explain the procedure and its purpose to your patient. Also, take this opportunity to teach your patient as much as possible about her colostomy.

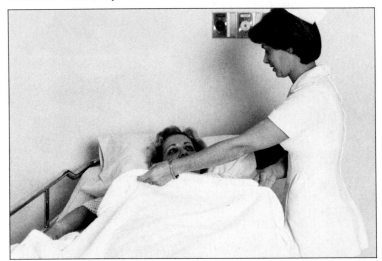

2 Fasten one end of the belt to the gasket on the ir-rigator drain. Twist the belt into posi-tion, as the nurse is doing here.

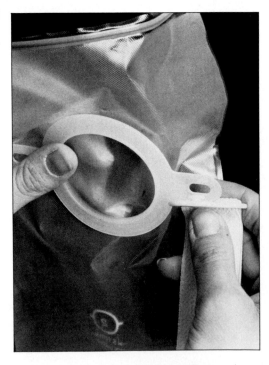

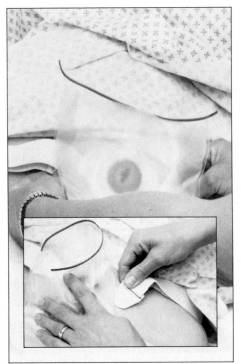

3 Next, place Ms. Johnson in a semi-Fowler's position. Then, use one hand to hold the gasket away from your patient's body as you use your other hand to wrap the belt around her waist. Place the belt's soft side against her skin, with the buttons facing away from her body.

Attach the other end of the belt to the gas-ket (see inset). Care-fully center the gasket around Ms. Johnson's stoma.

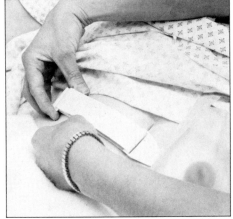

4 To check for tight-ness, slip your fingers between the belt and your patient's skin. A properly fitted belt will be snug around her waist. This prevents leakage during irrigation. If necessary, adjust the belt by moving the plastic adjuster, as shown here.

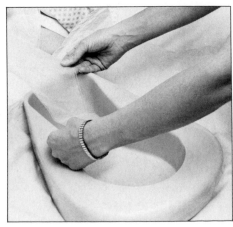

5 Set a bedpan next to Ms. Johnson. Tuck a bed-saver pad under the bedpan. Then, place the end of the irrigator drain into the bedpan.

When she's able, have your patient sit on the toilet, or on a chair next to the toilet, whichever she prefers. But, always make sure the bottom end of the irrigator drain hangs into the toilet.

6 Now, pull the tube out of the stoma cone, as shown here. Then, set it aside.
[Inset] Pop the disc off the cone by firmly squeezing the cone's sides.

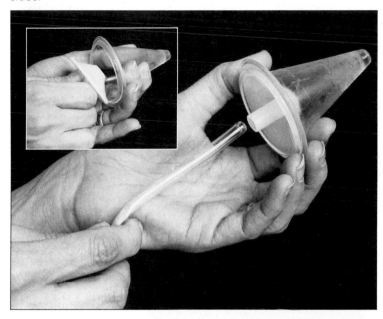

7 Push the cali-brated tube through the Stoma Seal disc. The disc's curved surfaces will face the tube's tip.
   Slide the disc along the tube until you reach the 3" (7.6 cm) mark indicated by Ms. Johnson's doc-tor.

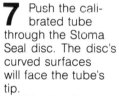
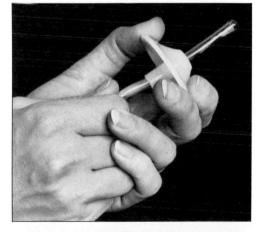

8 Next, gently twist together the end of the colon tube and the end of the tube leading to the irrigator, until you hear a snap.

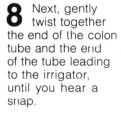
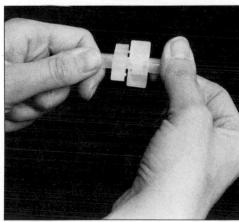

9 Check to be sure the irriga-tor's flow control is completely closed. Fill the irrigator with 1,000 ml warm tap water or irrigating solution, as ordered by the doctor.
   Hang the filled irrigator on an I.V. pole next to your patient's bed. Re-member, during the irrigation proce-dure, the bottom of the irrigator should be at your patient's shoulder level. If it isn't, adjust the height of the I.V. pole.

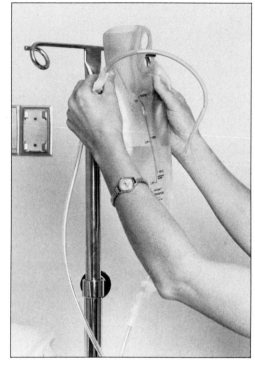

10 Hold the end of the colon tube over the bed-pan. Open the flow control and allow a small amount of water or irrigating solution to run through the tubing. This will force any trapped air out of the tubing. Clamp the flow control.

11 Next, open the package of water soluble lubricant. Squeeze a small amount onto a gauze pad or paper towel. Lubri-cate the first 3" (7.6 cm) of the tube.

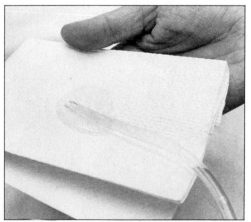

Stoma care

How to irrigate a colostomy continued

12 Now you're ready to insert the tube into your patient's stoma. Because this is the first time you're irrigating Ms. Johnson's colostomy, you need to know in which direction her intestine curves. As you know, you can't tell the curve of an intestine from a stoma location. To determine the curve, ask the doctor, or put on a finger cot and insert your little finger into your patient's stoma.

Then, slowly slide the colon tube into the open top of the irrigator drain, then through Ms. Johnson's stoma.

Suppose you meet resistance. Your patient may have impacted feces. To loosen the impaction, pull the tube out slightly, and unclamp the water flow control. Allow a small amount of water to flow into the intestine. Wait about 5 minutes for the water to soften the fecal matter. Then, try again. If several attempts to insert the tube fail, discontinue the procedure and notify the doctor.

Caution: Never force the tube into the intestine, because you may perforate the bowel.

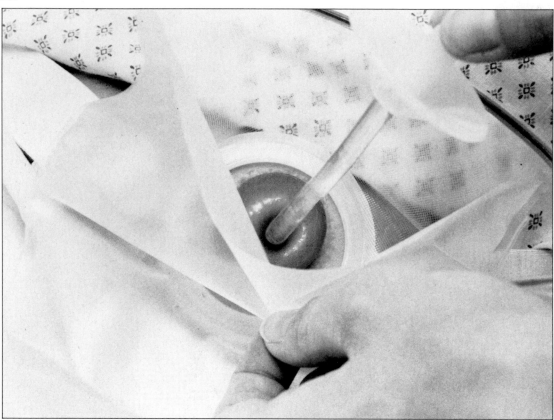

13 Using a stoma cone tip for irrigation reduces the risk of bowel perforation. If the doctor's asked you to use a stoma cone tip, proceed as follows. Insert the lubricated stoma cone through the open end of the irrigator drain, then into your patient's stoma. To prevent backflow, always hold the cone in place against the stoma.

Remember: Some doctors recommend dilating the stoma before inserting the stoma cone. However, *never* dilate your patient's stoma unless ordered by the doctor. For details on how to dilate a stoma, see page 101.

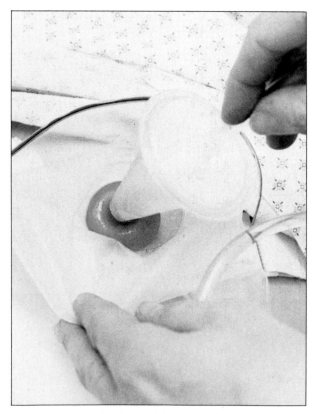

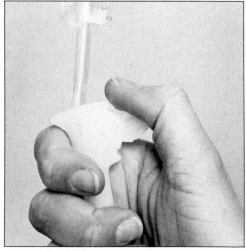

14 Open the flow clamp of the irrigator and slowly infuse the water or irrigating solution into your patient's colon.

If your patient complains of abdominal cramps, reduce or stop the infusion until the cramps subside. To do this, adjust the water flow control, or lower the irrigator bag.

☎ *Nursing tip:* To permit better fluid retention, allow the stoma cone or seal to remain in place for about 2 minutes after the infusion's complete.

15 Then, slowly remove the colon tube from Ms. Johnson's stoma, as the nurse is doing here.

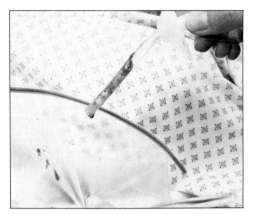

16 Now, close the irrigator drain by folding the blue closure strip outward and downward two times. Collect the initial irrigation return in the bed-pan, and note its appearance.

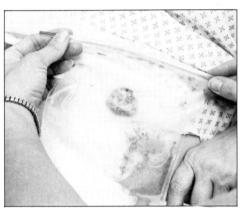

17 Clamp the bottom of the irrigator drain. After the initial return, it will take up to 30 minutes for the colon to empty completely. Encourage your patient to rest or engage in some other activity until her colon empties.
Nursing tip: A gentle abdominal massage may help speed up the return.

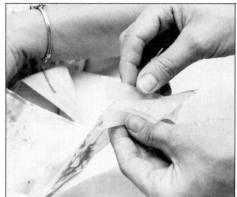

18 After all the irrigation has returned, unhook the belt and remove the irrigator drain. Clean the area around your patient's stoma with warm water. Dry the area thoroughly, and apply a clean colostomy pouch. Rinse and discard the irrigator drain.
    In your nurses' notes, document the procedure and any patient teaching you've given.

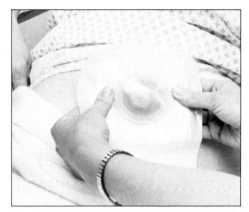

How to drain a continent ileostomy

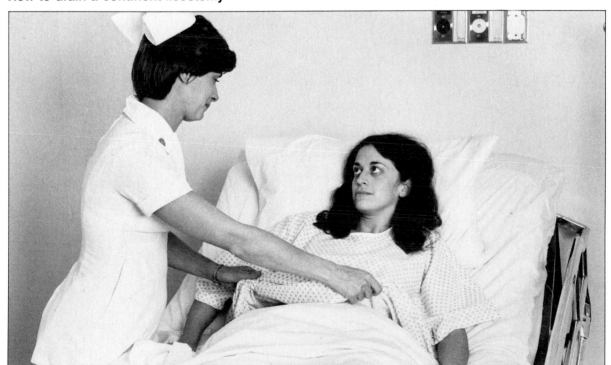

1 *Let's say Regina Simpson, a 32-year-old teacher, has had her colon removed because of cancer. During surgery, the doctor performed a continent ileos-tomy. He's left orders for you to drain the ileos-tomy every 2 hours. Here's the correct procedure:*
    To begin, assemble the following equipment: No. 28 catheter, water-soluble lubricant, bed-saver pad, bedpan, bulb syringe, warm tap water, and a gauze pad or stoma cap.
    Then, explain the pro-cedure to Ms. Simpson. Expose the area around her stoma.

Stoma care

How to drain a continent ileostomy continued

2 Next, place the bedpan on the bed next to Ms. Simpson. Tuck the bed-saver pad underneath the pan. (When she's able, your patient can perform the procedure in the bathroom, draining the catheter directly into the toilet.)

Now, squeeze a small amount of lubricant onto the gauze pad. Apply the lubricant to the catheter tip. Place the other end of the catheter in the bedpan.

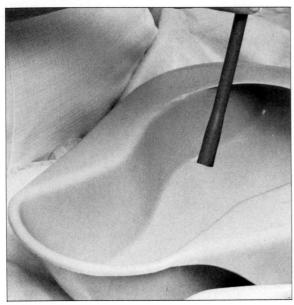

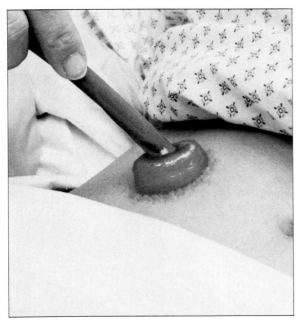

3 Carefully insert the lubricated end of the catheter into Ms. Simpson's stoma. When the catheter reaches the nipple valve, you'll feel resistance.

At this point, ask your patient to take a deep breath. As she does, gently push the catheter through the nipple valve. Then, tell your patient to resume normal breathing.

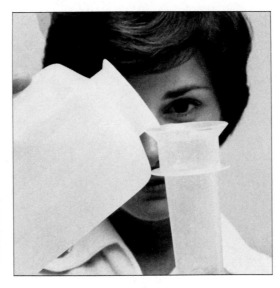

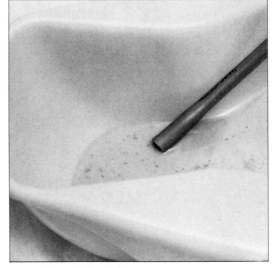

4 If you still meet resistance, try this method:

Fill a bulb syringe with 40 ml warm tap water. Remove the open end of the catheter from the bedpan. Hold the end upright so the water doesn't flow out. Insert the syringe tip in the catheter and slowly infuse the water. As you do this, try passing the catheter through the nipple valve.

When the catheter passes through the nipple valve, stop the infusion. Then, remove the bulb syringe and return the open end of the catheter to the bedpan.

If you continue to meet resistance, notify the doctor.

5 When the drainage begins flowing into the bedpan, you'll know the catheter has passed into your patient's ileostomy reservoir. Check the drainage. If it looks very thick, the doctor may instruct you to use a bulb syringe to infuse 30 to 40 ml water into the reservoir. This will dilute the drainage.

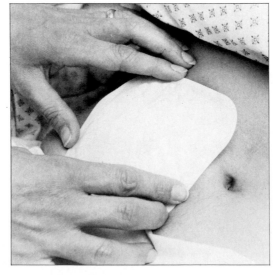

6 As soon as the drainage stops, gently remove the catheter from Ms. Simpson's stoma. Then, clean her stoma with warm tap water, and dry it thoroughly.

Next, place a gauze pad or a stoma cap over her stoma. Wash the catheter with warm water.

Document the procedure in your nurses' notes.

Home care

How to empty your ostomy pouch

1

Dear Patient:
The nurse has shown you how to empty your ostomy pouch while you're in the hospital. Here are some guidelines to help you empty your pouch in your bathroom at home.

As you know, you'll empty your ostomy pouch when it's about one third full. If you have a colostomy, the pouch will usually need to be emptied once or twice daily. You'll probably have to empty an ileostomy pouch five or six times daily.

To prepare for the procedure, place a cup of warm water within reach. Then, sit on the toilet with the pouch hanging between your legs.

2

Or, if you prefer, sit on a chair next to the toilet. But, be sure the pouch's opening is in the toilet.

3

Now you're ready to empty your pouch. To do this, turn up the bottom of the pouch and remove the closure clamp.

To prevent splashing, place some toilet paper on the surface of the water, or flush the toilet as you point the pouch's unclamped opening into the bowl.

4

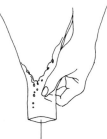

Slide your thumb and index finger down the outside of the pouch, squeezing all the contents into the toilet.

5

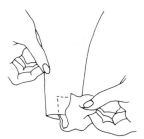

Next, use tissue or a disposable wipe to clean any remaining drainage from outside and inside the pouch opening.

6

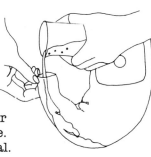

Hold the pouch opening upright and pour the cup of water into the pouch, as shown here. Swish the water around to remove any remaining drainage. As you work, avoid wetting your stoma or the pouch adhesive. Doing so could break the seal.

7

Now, direct the pouch opening into the toilet. Let the pouch drain thoroughly.

If you use a pouch deodorant, place it in the pouch, following the manufacturer's directions. Then, using a clean disposable wipe or toilet tissue, clean and dry the outside of the pouch. Finally, close the pouch with a clamp or rubber band.

Patient teaching

Home care

How to clean a reusable pouch

1

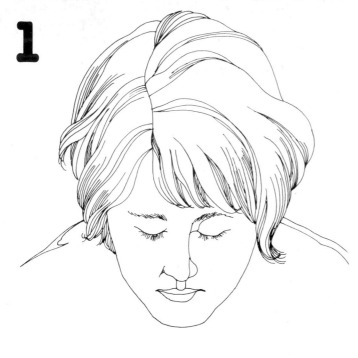

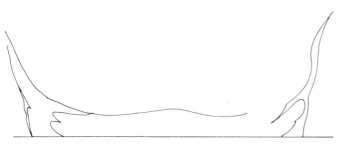

Dear Patient:
To increase the life of your reusable pouch and help prevent odor, clean your pouch thoroughly every time you change it. Having at least two pouches is advisable. This way you can clean one while you're wearing the other.

Here's how to clean your pouch:

First, remove the double-adhesive disc from the faceplate. If you can't remove all of the adhesive, try rolling the rest of it off with your fingertips.

2

Or, try loosening the adhesive with a gauze pad moistened in adhesive solvent. But, remember, always use solvent sparingly. Too much solvent may erode the faceplate.

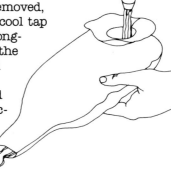

3

After the adhesive's removed, rinse the pouch with cool tap water. Then, using a long-handled brush, scrub the inside with water and a mild soap or detergent (as recommended by the pouch manufacturer).

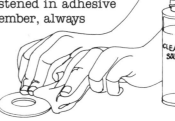

4

Rinse the bag thoroughly with cool water. Then, fill the pouch with wadded paper towels and place it on a flat surface to dry.

Or use a pouch hook to hang it over your sink.

Important: Never dry a pouch in direct sunlight or heat.

When the pouch is completely dry, remove the paper towels, if you've used any. Store the pouch in a cool, dry place.

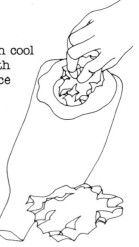

Stoma care

Administering medication to an ostomy patient

Planning to administer medication to your ostomy patient? If so, you'll want to take certain measures to make sure the medication's absorbed properly.

As you know, most oral medications are absorbed through the upper intestinal lining. But, suppose your patient's an ostomate with an irritated or shortened upper intestinal tract. Some oral medications, such as enteric coated tablets and sustained-released capsules, may not be totally absorbed in the intestinal lining.

Suppose your patient's medication isn't being absorbed. Check with the doctor to see if his medication's available in a liquid preparation or uncoated tablet. If it isn't, ask the doctor if the medication can be given by another route, such as I.V. or I.M. *Note:* To aid absorption, some tablets can be crushed prior to administration.

If your patient takes a new oral medication, either you or he should feel his pouch for pills or capsules before emptying it. Also, remind him that oral medication may affect the color and consistency of his drainage. For example, an antacid may make his drainage appear white and pasty.

Here are some additional considerations to review with your patient:
• Some vitamin preparations cause unpleasant pouch odor, particularly in rubber pouches. As a precaution, suggest that your patient wear an old pouch or use a disposable pouch when taking a vitamin for the first time. Then, if the vitamin causes an odor, have him wear an old pouch or a disposable pouch every time he takes it.
• Laxatives and diuretics may cause dehydration and should not be taken without an order.
• Warn your patient *never* to allow anyone to give him a rectal enema, unless ordered by the doctor. Even if his rectum's intact following surgery, an enema may damage the remaining tissue.

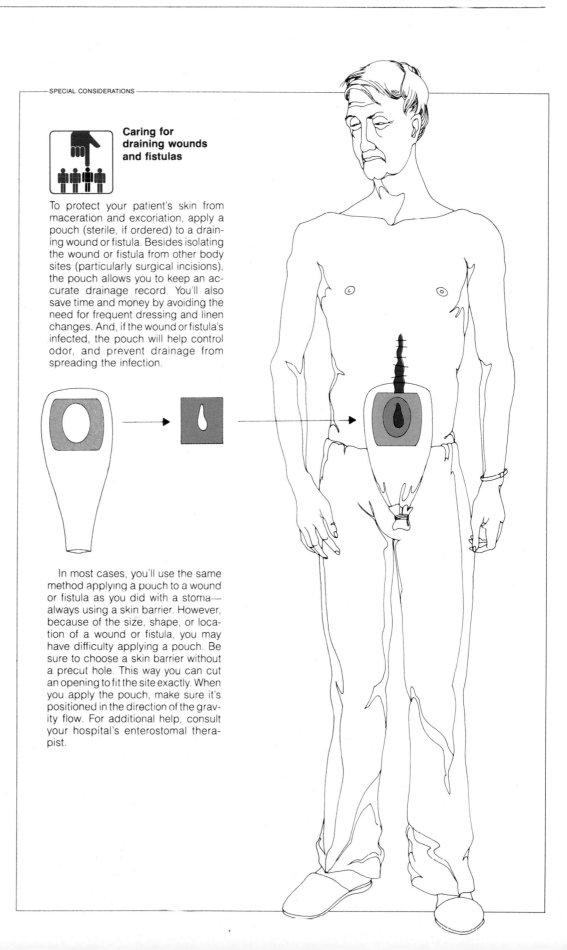

Caring for draining wounds and fistulas

To protect your patient's skin from maceration and excoriation, apply a pouch (sterile, if ordered) to a draining wound or fistula. Besides isolating the wound or fistula from other body sites (particularly surgical incisions), the pouch allows you to keep an accurate drainage record. You'll also save time and money by avoiding the need for frequent dressing and linen changes. And, if the wound or fistula's infected, the pouch will help control odor, and prevent drainage from spreading the infection.

In most cases, you'll use the same method applying a pouch to a wound or fistula as you did with a stoma—always using a skin barrier. However, because of the size, shape, or location of a wound or fistula, you may have difficulty applying a pouch. Be sure to choose a skin barrier without a precut hole. This way you can cut an opening to fit the site exactly. When you apply the pouch, make sure it's positioned in the direction of the gravity flow. For additional help, consult your hospital's enterostomal therapist.

Intestinal tube care

Sooner or later, you'll care for a patient who needs an intestinal tube. Do you know how to assist the doctor with the insertion? How to verify proper tube placement? Or what to do if your patient starts gagging during insertion?

Learn more about intestinal tubes by reading this section. We'll explain:
• how to insert a double- or single-lumen tube.
• how to administer a tube feeding.
• how to withdraw mercury from a single-lumen tube.
• how to test the tube's balloon for leaks.

Nurses' guide to intestinal tubes

Chances are, you're familiar with the various types of intestinal tubes. But, do you know how to assist the doctor in the insertion of a Miller-Abbott tube? Or how to insert a feeding tube? Study this chart for the answers.

Remember: No matter which tube's inserted into your patient, you must provide good mouth care, and check his nostrils frequently for signs of irritation. If you see any signs of irritation, retape the tube so it doesn't cause tension. Then, lubricate the nostril. Or, check with the doctor to see if the tube can be inserted through the other nostril.

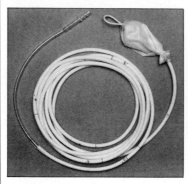

Kaslow® radiopaque

Description
• Ten-foot long (3m), single-lumen, rubber tube with centimeter markings. Available in size 16 French

Use
• For bowel obstruction: When attached to intermittent suction, allows aspiration of intestinal contents.

Nursing considerations
• Be prepared to assist doctor with insertion.
• Place patient in high Fowler's position with his neck hyperextended.
• Before insertion, test tube for patency and balloon for leaks.
• Attach to intermittent low suction, as ordered.
• Once every 8 hours (or as ordered), document type and amount of drainage.

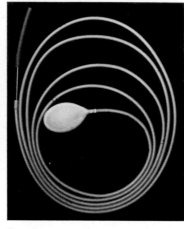

Cantor

Description
• Ten-foot long (3 m), single-lumen, rubber tube with balloon at distal tip for mercury insertion. Available in size 16 French

Use
• For bowel obstruction: When attached to suction, allows aspiration of intestinal contents.

Nursing considerations
• Be prepared to assist doctor with tube insertion.
• Place patient in high Fowler's position with his neck hyperextended.
• Before insertion, test tube for patency and balloon for leaks.
• Insert mercury into balloon.
• Attach suction lumen to intermittent suction, as ordered.
• Once every 8 hours (or as ordered), document type and amount of drainage.

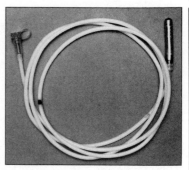

Dobbhoff™ enteric feeding tube

Description
• A 45″ (114 cm), Erythrothane® polyurethane, radiopaque, single-lumen tube with mercury-filled bolus at the tip

Use
• Allows continuous intestinal feeding.

Nursing considerations
• Insert only as ordered by doctor.
• Position patient in high Fowler's position with neck erect.
• Initially insert two thirds of tube into the stomach. Advance remainder of tube at a rate of 2 to 3 inches (5 to 7.6 cm) per hour. Weighted mercury bolus helps advance tube to small intestine.
• Before starting tube feeding, determine tube's placement using tests on page 52.
• Be sure feeding solution is at room temperature, to avoid cramps or diarrhea.
• Administer water as initial tube feeding, for 2 to 4 hours or until patient's tolerance to tube and infusion is noted.
• Start half-strength solution tube feedings at a rate of 25 ml an hour, or as ordered. Increase to full-strength solution within 24 hours.
• Never use an infusion pump that delivers more than 40 pounds per square inch (psi) of pressure. The tube's bursting strength is 80 psi. Also, when irrigating tube, use only a 50 cc syringe. Excessive pressure from a smaller syringe may cause tube rupture.
• Watch patient for signs of feeding solution intolerance: nausea, vomiting, and diarrhea. If you see any of the above, stop the infusion and notify the doctor. You may be infusing the solution too rapidly, the solution may be contaminated, or the patient may be sensitive to the feeding solution.

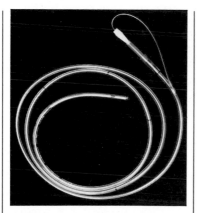

Hodge™ decompression tube

Description
- Double-lumen, 72″ or 96″ (183 or 244 cm) long tube with 4⅞″ long, mercury-weighted, radiopaque tip

Use
- When attached to suction, allows aspiration of intestinal contents.
- May be used to obtain intestinal, biliary, and pancreatic secretions for diagnostic tests.

Nursing considerations
- Insert tube only when ordered by doctor.
- Tube may be inserted nasally or orally for aspiration.
- Place patient in a low Fowler's position (30°).
- Initially, insert tube to stomach (around 50 cm).
- Have patient remain in right side-lying position during tube advancement.
- Advance tube 2 to 3 inches (5 to 7.6 cm) every hour, until tube reaches prescribed distance (75 cm, or as ordered).
- Aspirate tube contents. Presence of bile verifies tube position in duodenum.
- Attach suction lumen to intermittent suction, as ordered.
- Irrigate with 30 ml normal saline solution every 2 hours, as ordered.
- Inject 5 cc air into vent lumen to clear air vent. Never irrigate vent lumen with fluid.

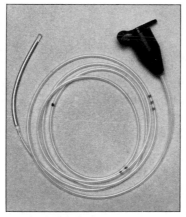

Keofeed® silicone-rubber

Description
- A 36″ (91 cm) silicone-rubber tube with centimeter markings (25, 50, 75 cm). Weighted at distal end with mercury bolus

Use
- Primarily used for gastric or intestinal feeding
- May be inserted through gastrostomy tube for continuous intestinal feeding.

Nursing considerations
- Insert tube only when ordered by doctor.
- Before inserting tube, lubricate Keofeed monofilament guide and advance through tube.
- Be sure tube feeding solution is at room temperature to help prevent cramps or diarrhea.
- Before starting tube feeding, determine tube's placement, using test on page 52.
- Administer water as initial feeding, for 2 to 4 hours or until patient's tolerance to tube and infusion noted.
- Start half-strength tube feedings at a rate of 25 ml an hour, or as ordered. Increase to full-strength solution within 24 hours.
- Watch patient for signs of feeding solution intolerance: nausea, vomiting and diarrhea. If you see any of the above, stop the infusion and notify the doctor. You may be infusing the solution too rapidly, the solution may be contaminated, or the patient may be sensitive to the feeding solution

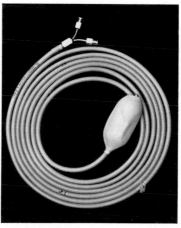

Miller-Abbott

Description
- Ten-foot long (3 m), double-lumen rubber tube with centimeter markings. Available in sizes 12, 14, 16, or 18 French

Use
- For bowel obstruction: When attached to suction, allows aspiration of intestinal contents.
- Dilates bowel.

Nursing considerations
- Be prepared to assist doctor with tube insertion.
- Place patient in high Fowler's position with head erect.
- Before insertion, test tube for patency and balloon for leaks.
- Insert mercury after tube reaches stomach.
- Attach suction lumen to intermittent suction, as ordered.
- Place syringe or clamp over balloon lumen to prevent accidental mercury withdrawal through suction.
- Once every 8 hours (or as ordered), document type and amount of drainage.

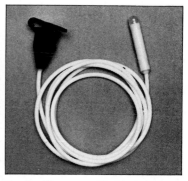

Keofeed® mercury bolus tube

Description
- A 43″ (109 cm), radiopaque, silicone-rubber tube with centimeter markings (25, 50, 75 cm). Weighted at distal end with 5 gram mercury bolus

Use
- Used for gastric or intestinal feeding

Nursing considerations
- Insert tube only when ordered by doctor.
- Before inserting tube, lubricate Keofeed monofilament guide and advance it through tube.
- Place patient in high Fowler's position with his neck hyperextended.
- Before insertion, test tube for patency and balloon for leaks.
- Tell patient to remain in right side-lying position during tube advancement.
- Insert tube to premeasured mark for gastric feeding. Advance 2 to 3 inches (5 to 7.6 cm) per hour to 75 cm mark (or, as ordered) for intestinal feeding. Weighted bolus helps advance tube to small intestine.
- Before starting tube feeding, determine tube position with tests described on page 52.
- Administer water as initial tube feeding, for 2 to 4 hours or until patient's tolerance to tube and infusion is noted.
- Start half-strength solution tube feedings at a rate of 25 ml an hour, or as ordered. Increase to full-strength solution within 24 hours.
- Watch patient for signs of feeding solution intolerance: nausea, vomiting, and diarrhea. If you see any of the above, stop the infusion and notify the doctor. You may be infusing the solution too rapidly, the solution may be contaminated, or the patient may be sensitive to the feeding solution.

Intestinal tube care

Inserting a single-lumen intestinal tube

1 *How familiar are you with single-lumen intestinal tubes? Do you know how to assist the doctor with an insertion? If you're unsure, follow these steps:*

First, gather the necessary equipment: single-lumen tube (we'll use a Cantor tube), water-soluble lubricant, bed-saver pad, towel, 5 ml of mercury, 5 cc syringe with a 21-gauge needle, cotton-tipped applicator, drinking water with straw (or ice chips), water to test balloon patency, tissues, emesis basin, tincture of benzoin or Skin-Prep, and nonallergenic tape.

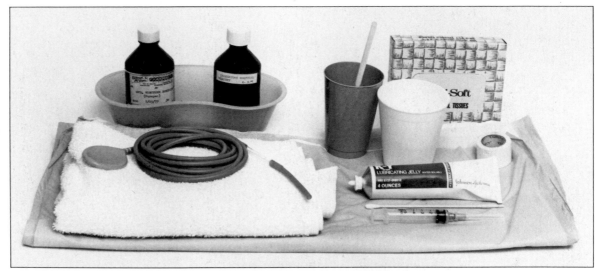

2 Now, test the tube's patency by running water through it. Then, check the tube's balloon for leaks.

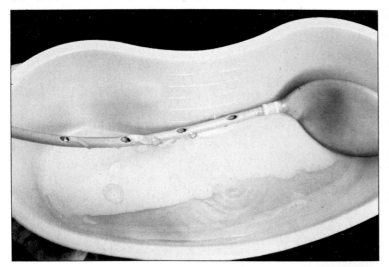

3 To do this, inject 10 cc of air into the balloon with a 10 cc syringe and 21-gauge needle. Then, immerse the balloon in water and watch for air bubbles. If none are present, the balloon's okay. Remove the balloon from the water.

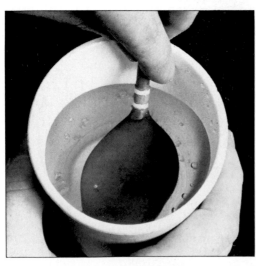

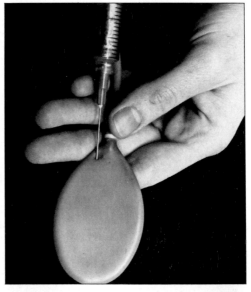

4 Using a 5 cc syringe with a 21-gauge needle, draw up the mercury. Inject the mercury into the upper portion of the bag, holding the needle in place, as shown here. The mercury will flow to the base of the balloon.

Then, with the needle above the level of the mercury, aspirate all the air, collapsing the balloon. Remove the needle from the balloon.

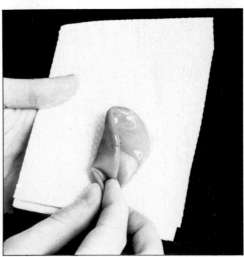

5 Generously lubricate the first 6" (15.2 cm) of the tube with water-soluble lubricant.

6 Now, prepare your patient for the procedure. Warn her that it will be uncomfortable. Agree on a special signal she can use to tell you or the doctor to stop for a moment; for example, raising her hand, or tapping her arm.

Seat your patient upright in bed. Cover her gown with the bed-saver pad or a towel, to protect it from spills (see photo). Then, hyperextend your patient's neck.

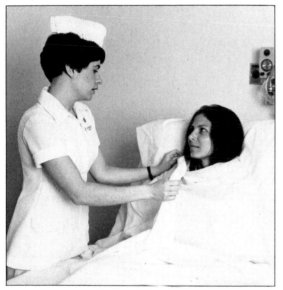

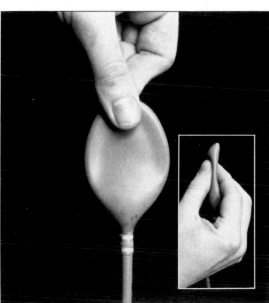

7 After the doctor's determined how much tube to insert, he'll be ready to begin the procedure. Ask your patient to hold her head still.

The doctor will hold the end of the catheter upward so the mercury drops to the base of the balloon, as shown here.

To keep the mercury at the base, the doctor will pinch the balloon closed (see inset).

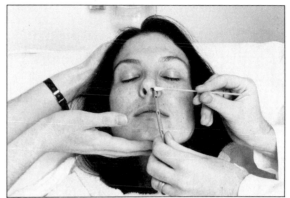

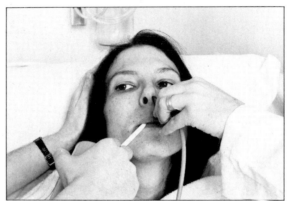

8 Then, the doctor will slowly begin inserting the tube into your patient's nostril. When the tip of the tube's in the nostril, he'll release the balloon, allowing the mercury to flow to the other end. (This will help pull the balloon down into the nasopharynx.) He'll then use a long cotton-tipped applicator to help advance the balloon into the laryngopharynx.

Throughout the procedure, continue to reassure your patient.

9 As the doctor advances the tube into your patient's laryngopharynx, your patient may begin to gag. If that happens, the doctor will stop advancing the tube to prevent your patient from vomiting. To relax the patient's laryngopharynx, instruct her to take several deep breaths. Or, if she is allowed to drink water, ask her to take sips of water through the straw. Reassure your patient before continuing.

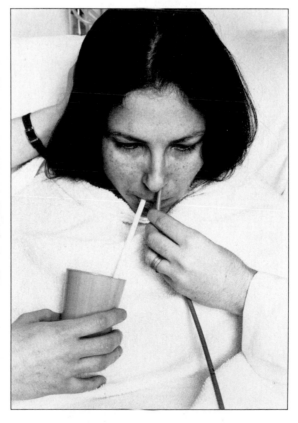

10 Now, the doctor will be ready to advance the tube into the esophagus and stomach. To make the procedure easier, ask your patient to place her chin on her chest and continue to sip water or chew ice chips.

🔹 *Nursing tip:* If your patient can't drink water, have her dry-swallow at the doctor's signal.

The doctor will advance the tube 3″ to 5″ (7.6 to 12.7 cm) each time your patient swallows, until the tube reaches your patient's stomach. Then, he'll check proper tube placement, secure the tube, and continue to advance the tube into your patient's intestine (see pages 116 and 117 for details).

Document the procedure in your nurses' notes.

Intestinal tube care

Inserting a double-lumen intestinal tube

1 *Let's assume Terry Monroe, a 35-year-old chemist, has been admitted to your unit with a bowel obstruction. The doctor has decided to insert a double-lumen intestinal tube. (In this story, we'll be using a Miller-Abbott tube.) Here's how to assist:*

Begin by gathering the equipment you'll need: double-lumen intestinal tube, water-soluble lubricant, bed-saver pad, towel, cotton-tipped applicator, mercury (if ordered), non-allergenic tape, drinking water with straw (or ice chips), water to test balloon patency, 5 cc syringe with a 21-gauge needle, tissues, emesis basin, and tincture of benzoin or Skin-Prep.

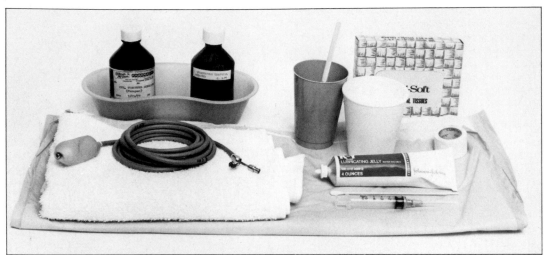

2 Run water through the tube to check its patency.

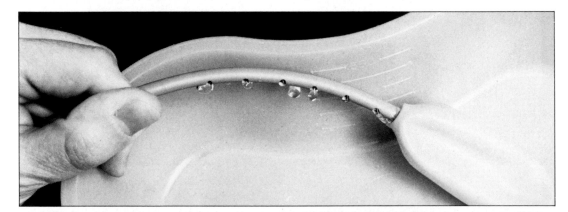

3 Next, test the tube's balloon for holes or cuts, which could allow mercury to escape into your patient's intestine. To do this, inject 5 cc air into the balloon lumen.

[Inset] Keeping the syringe in place, immerse the balloon in the container of water, as shown here. If air bubbles appear, assume the balloon has a leak and replace the tube. If no air bubbles appear, remove the balloon from the water. Disconnect the syringe, releasing the air from the balloon.

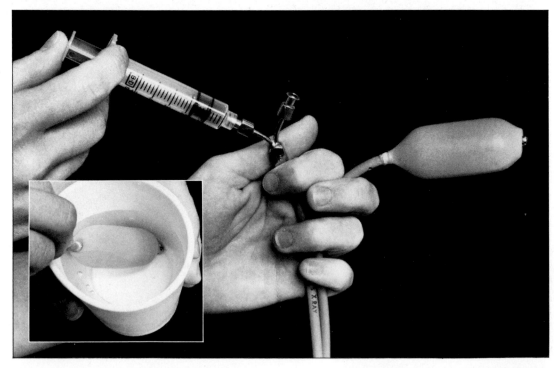

4 Now, tell your patient what you're going to do, and warn her that the procedure will be uncomfortable. Agree on a special signal she can use to tell you or the doctor to stop for a moment, such as raising her hand or tapping your arm.

Important: Is your patient extremely anxious? If so, the doctor may want a sedative administered I.V. before starting the procedure.

Place Ms. Monroe in a high Fowler's position. Then, put a bed-saver pad or a towel across her gown to protect it from spills. Give her a handful of tissues, because intubation may cause tearing. Place an emesis basin within her reach.

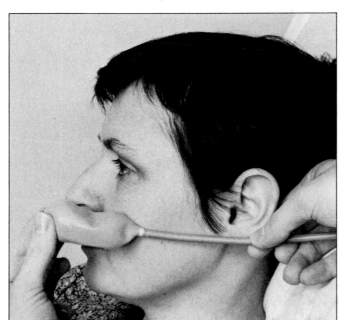

6 Then, he'll measure the distance between your patient's earlobe and her midsternum. He'll total these measurements—usually it totals about 55" (140 cm)—and mark the tube correspondingly.

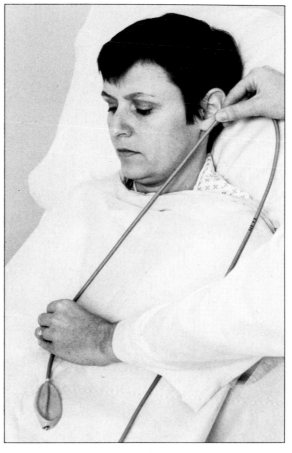

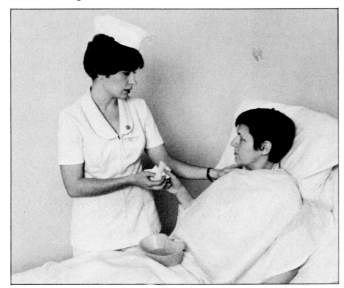

5 The doctor will determine how much tube to insert. To do this, he'll first estimate the distance to your patient's stomach. Using the tube, he'll measure the distance from Ms. Monroe's earlobe to the tip of her nose, as shown here.

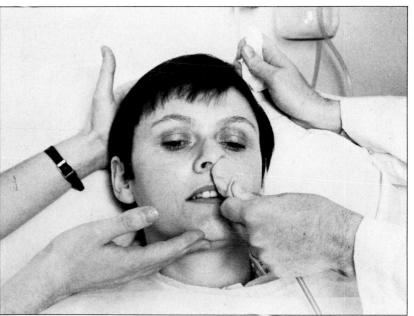

7 Now, apply water-soluble lubricant to the first 6" (15.2 cm) of the tube.
Note: Never lubricate an intestinal tube with petroleum jelly.

Next, ask your patient to hold her head erect so the doctor can begin the insertion, as shown here.

Intestinal tube care

Inserting a double-lumen intestinal tube continued

8 When the tube reaches Ms. Monroe's laryngopharynx, she may gag. To prevent vomiting, the doctor will stop advancing the tube.

Help your patient calm the gag reflex by telling her to take several deep breaths. If she's allowed to drink water, ask her to take short sips of water through the straw. Then, wait a few moments before continuing.

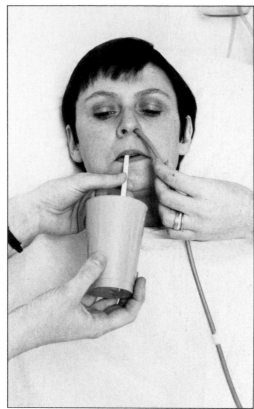

9 Now, ask your patient to tilt her head slightly forward. This will close her trachea and open up her esophagus. To keep your patient from gagging during this part of the procedure, instruct her to sip water through the straw, or to suck on ice chips.

Nursing tip: If your patient isn't allowed to drink water, ask her to dry-swallow at the doctor's signal.

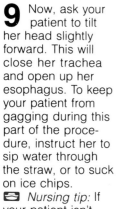

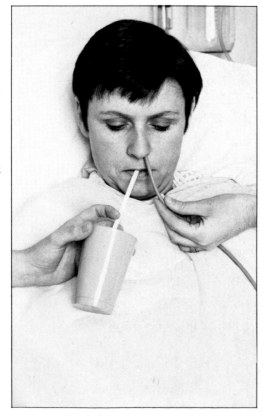

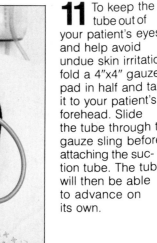

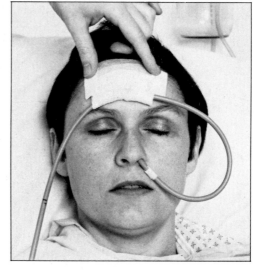

10 After the doctor determines the tube's in your patient's stomach, he'll infuse 2 to 5 ml of mercury into the balloon lumen. He'll keep a syringe on this lumen as long as the tube is in place to prevent accidental suctioning of the mercury.

11 To keep the tube out of your patient's eyes and help avoid undue skin irritation, fold a 4"x4" gauze pad in half and tape it to your patient's forehead. Slide the tube through the gauze sling before attaching the suction tube. The tube will then be able to advance on its own.

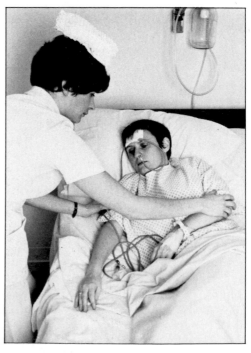

12 To make it easier to advance the tube into her intestine, position Ms. Monroe on her right side. Explain she'll remain in this position until the tube reaches the desired position.

13 Every hour, slowly advance the tube 2″ to 3″ (5 to 7.6 cm), until it reaches the premeasured mark, or as ordered by the doctor. Gravity and peristalsis will help advance the tube. Be sure to keep the 4″ (10.2 cm) of the tube that's outside of the nose well lubricated to help ease passage and prevent irritation.

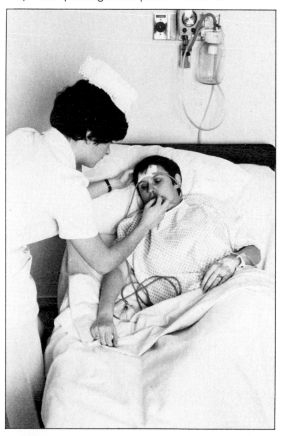

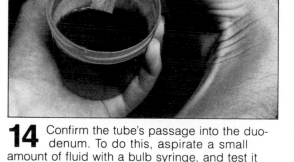

14 Confirm the tube's passage into the duodenum. To do this, aspirate a small amount of fluid with a bulb syringe, and test it with litmus paper to determine pH. If the tube's properly placed, the paper will turn blue, indicating an alkaline fluid.

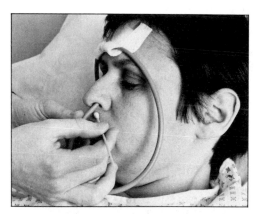

15 When you have advanced the tube to its proper place (usually confirmed by X-ray), secure it. To do this, apply Skin-Prep or tincture of benzoin (with a cotton-tipped applicator), under Ms. Monroe's nostril, as shown here. When the benzoin (or Skin-Prep) feels tacky, tape the tube over it.

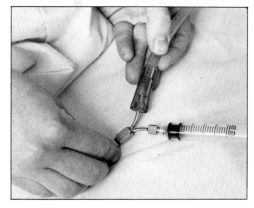

16 When you know the tube's properly placed in the intestine, attach the tube to intermittent low suction, or as ordered by the doctor.

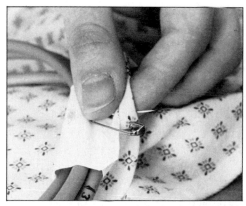

17 If you have a considerable length of tube remaining, coil it and wrap it with tape, leaving a tab at one end. Then, safety-pin the tab to her gown, just below shoulder level (see photo).

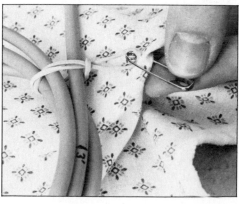

18 As an alternative, loop a rubber band around the tube, as shown here. Then, pin the rubber band to your patient's gown.
 Finally, document the entire procedure in your notes.
 To help your patient remain as comfortable as possible, provide good mouth care. Tell her to brush her teeth regularly. Also, routinely check your patient to make sure the tube's positioned properly.

Intestinal tube care

How to remove an intestinal tube

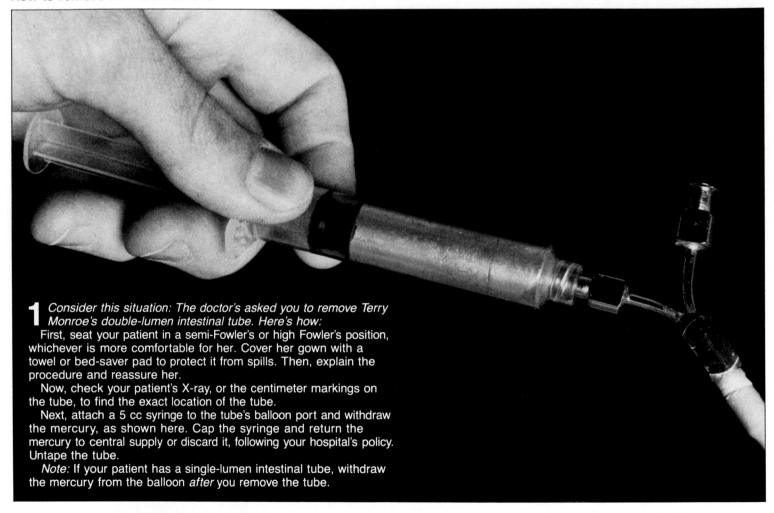

1 *Consider this situation: The doctor's asked you to remove Terry Monroe's double-lumen intestinal tube. Here's how:*
First, seat your patient in a semi-Fowler's or high Fowler's position, whichever is more comfortable for her. Cover her gown with a towel or bed-saver pad to protect it from spills. Then, explain the procedure and reassure her.
Now, check your patient's X-ray, or the centimeter markings on the tube, to find the exact location of the tube.
Next, attach a 5 cc syringe to the tube's balloon port and withdraw the mercury, as shown here. Cap the syringe and return the mercury to central supply or discard it, following your hospital's policy. Untape the tube.
Note: If your patient has a single-lumen intestinal tube, withdraw the mercury from the balloon *after* you remove the tube.

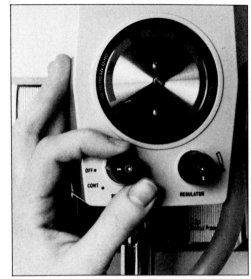

2 Is the tube attached to a suction machine? If so, turn the machine off before proceeding further.

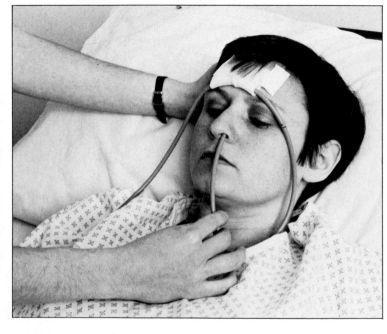

3 Now, slowly withdraw about 6″ to 8″ (15.2 to 20.3 cm) of the tube, as the nurse is doing here. Wait 10 minutes. Then, withdraw another 6″ to 8″. Wait 10 minutes more.
Continue this procedure until the end of the tube reaches your patient's esophagus. At this point, about 18″ (45 cm) of the tube will still be in place.

4 Ms. Monroe's tube is already connected to the suction machine. But if your patient's tube isn't, connect it. Now, turn on the suction machine. When the tube's clear, turn off the machine.

Now, you're ready to withdraw the tube. To prevent your patient from aspirating any remaining fluid, pinch the end of the tubing.

[Inset] Or, fold over the end of the tube and hold it securely, as shown.

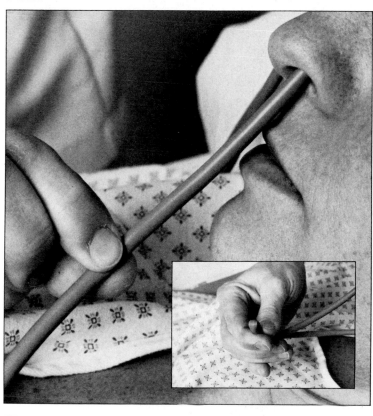

6 Suppose your patient has a single-lumen tube, such as a Cantor tube. You'll remove the mercury from the balloon, using a 21-gauge needle and syringe (see photo). Return the mercury to central supply, or dispose of it, according to hospital policy.

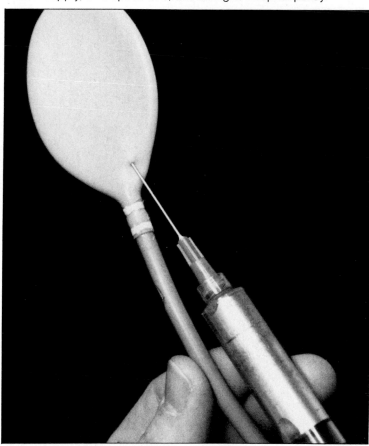

5 Tell Ms. Monroe to take a deep breath and hold it. As she does this, quickly remove the tube. If you meet resistance, notify the doctor. Never forcibly remove a tube.

When you're finished, ask Ms. Monroe to breathe normally.

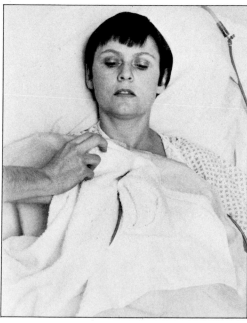

7 When you've removed the tube, clean your patient's nostrils. Place a small amount of water-soluble lubricant in each nostril. Provide proper mouth care, including a gargle.

If your patient's tube is disposable, throw it away. If it isn't, clean the tube and return it to central supply for sterilization.

Finally, document the procedure in your nurses' notes.

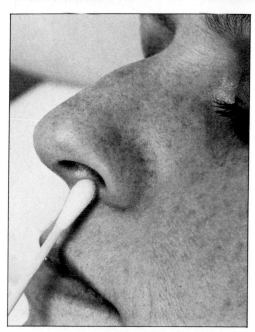

Intestinal tube care

Inserting an intestinal tube via gastrostomy tube

1 *Suppose the doctor orders intestinal tube feeding for a patient in your unit. The patient already has a gastrostomy tube in place, but you'll need to insert an intestinal tube. Will you know what to do? If you're unsure, read this photostory.*

Gather the following equipment: intestinal tube (we're using a Keofeed silicone-rubber feeding tube with a mercury-weighted tip); water-soluble lubricant; Keofeed monofilament guide; paper towel; and a 3 cc syringe.

Note: Be sure to choose a feeding tube that's small enough to fit through the gastrostomy tube.

Explain the procedure to your patient. Ask him to lie flat and place a bedsaver pad under his left side.

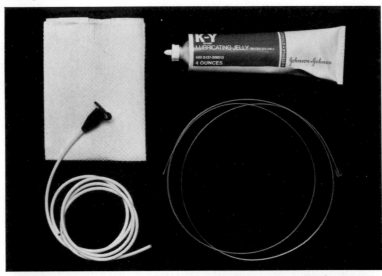

2 Squeeze a small amount of lubricant into a medicine cup. Then, using the syringe, draw up 2 to 3 ml of lubricant.

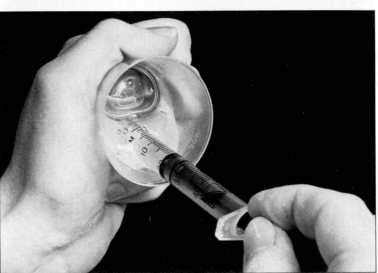

3 Now, inject the lubricant into the feeding tube adapter, as shown here. Carefully insert the monofilament as far as it will go (see inset).

Caution: During the insertion, take care not to puncture the side of the tube or push the guide through a feeding port.

Close the adapter cap to keep the guide from slipping out.

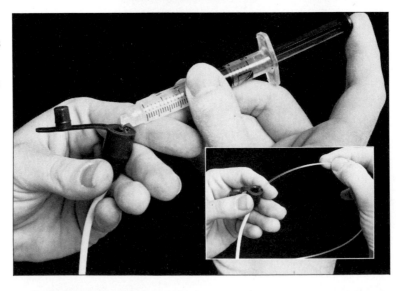

4 Now you're ready to insert the feeding tube. Lubricate the first 12″ (30 cm) of the tube.

Hold up your patient's gastrostomy tube to prevent leakage of the tube's contents. Then, unclamp the tube.

5 Gently advance the lubricated end of the feeding tube through the entire length of the gastrostomy tube, about 10″ to 12″ (25 to 30 cm).

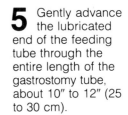

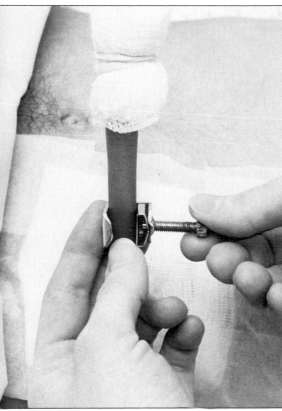

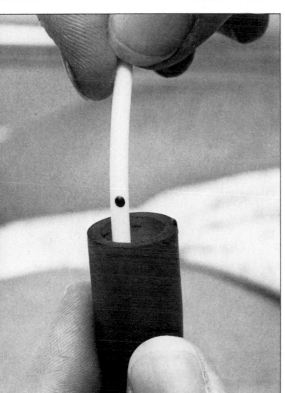

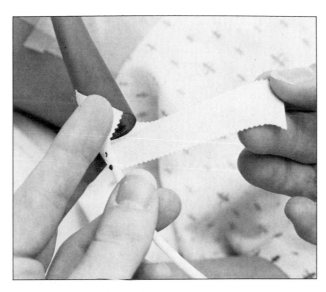

6 Now, tape the end of the feeding tube to the gastrostomy tube to keep it in place.

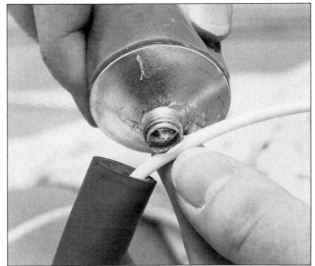

7 Turn your patient onto his right side, where he'll remain for 2 to 4 hours. Keep the distal part of the tube clamped.

Tell your patient this right side-lying position will allow the tube to pass more easily into his small intestine.

Now, remove the tape from the tubes and lubricate the feeding tube. Then, slowly advance it ½" (1.3 cm) every 15 minutes, until you reach the distance ordered by the doctor. (Make sure this is confirmed by X-ray.)

Securely tape the feeding and gastrostomy tubes together.

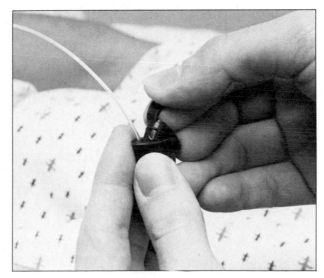
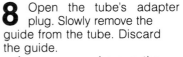

8 Open the tube's adapter plug. Slowly remove the guide from the tube. Discard the guide.

As soon as you're sure the tube's properly positioned, begin tube feedings, as ordered.

Finally, document the procedure in your nurses' notes.

Intestinal tube care

Continuous intestinal feeding using a volumetric pump

1 *Let's say your patient has an intestinal feeding tube in place. The doctor orders you to start continuous tube feeding at a rate of 50 ml an hour. To ensure an accurate infusion rate, you've decided to use a volumetric pump. (In this story the nurse will be using an Imed® 960 pump.) Do you know the correct procedure? If you're unsure, read these steps carefully.*

First, gather your equipment: prepared feeding solution, as ordered by the doctor; feeding bag (we're using a Dobbhoff bag); volumetric pump with Accuset® cassette and attached tubing; portable I.V. pole; and emesis basin.

Important: Never use a volumetric pump that delivers greater than 40 pounds per square inch (psi).

Then, explain the procedure to your patient. Make sure the feeding solution's at room temperature.

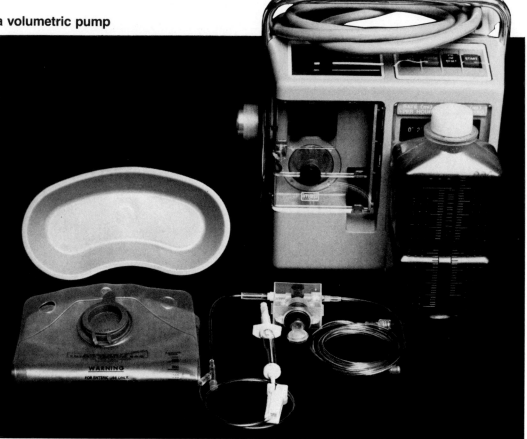

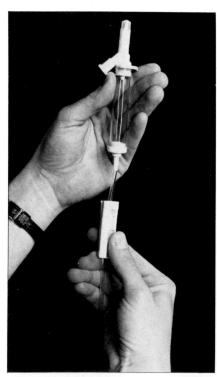

2 Now, slide the flow clamp along the tubing until it's under the drip chamber.

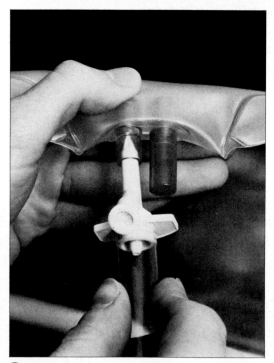

3 Next, remove the guard from the tubing spike, as well as the cap from the appropriate port at the bottom of the feeding bag. Grasping the bag firmly, insert the spike into it.

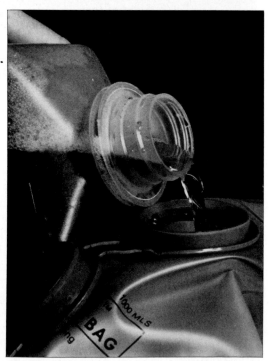

4 Open the cap at the top of the feeding bag and pour the feeding solution into the bag. Snap the cap closed. Then, hang the bag on the I.V. pole.

5 When that's done, squeeze the drip chamber until it's three quarters filled with the feeding solution.
Then, clamp the tube.

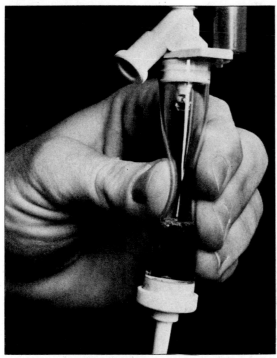

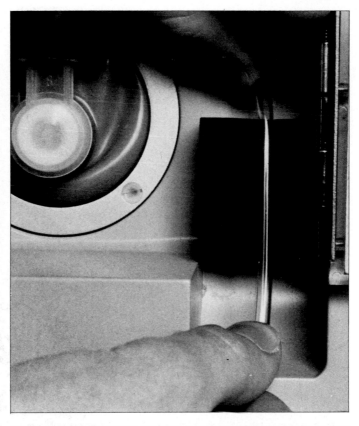

7 Slip the extension tubing into the air-in-line detector, as the nurse is doing here.
Now, close the door. If the door won't close, check the cassette and the tubing. Either may be positioned improperly.

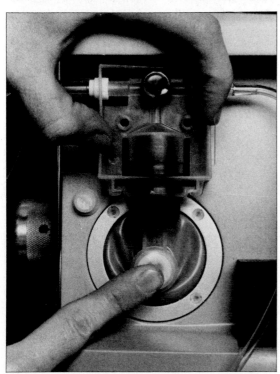

6 Now, open the clear plastic door and insert the cassette, as shown here. Then, snap the cassette plunger shaft into the locked position.

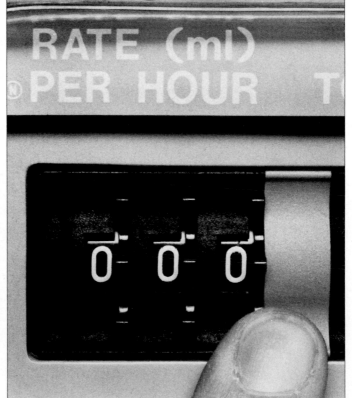

RATE (ml) PER HOUR

8 Unclamp the tubing and turn the RATE dial to 000. Also, set the VOLUME TO BE INFUSED dial at 0000.

Intestinal tube care

Continuous intestinal feeding using a volumetric pump continued

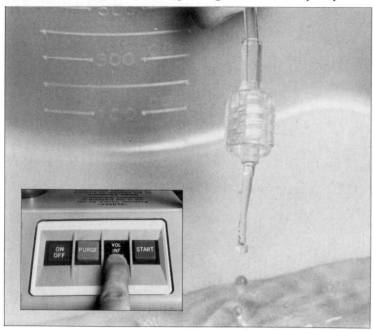

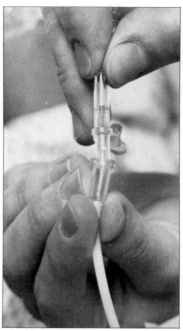

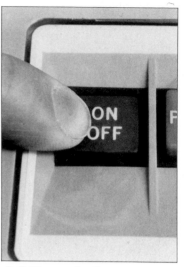

9 Turn on the pump and hold the cassette tubing over the basin. Press the pump's PURGE button until all the air is expelled from the tube.

Turn off the pump. Replace the protective cap and push the VOLUME INFUSED (VOL. INF.) RESET button (see inset). Set the RATE and VOLUME TO BE INFUSED dials, as ordered.

10 Confirm tube placement in your patient's intestine (see page 52). Then, remove the protective cap, and attach the cassette tubing to her intestinal tube.

11 Wrap adhesive tape around the connection to secure it.

Then, turn on the pump and pump alarms. Make sure the feeding solution is flowing continuously through the tubing. Check your patient frequently, making sure the RATE and VOLUME TO BE INFUSED dials are set properly.

12 Suppose your patient complains of abdominal cramps, or develops diarrhea. Stop the feeding immediately, and notify the doctor. Your patient may have an intestinal obstruction or a paralytic ileus.

To determine the cause of the problem, assess your patient's bowel sounds, as shown here, using guidelines given on page 23. If her bowel sounds are normal, the infusion's probably flowing too rapidly, or the patient can't tolerate tube feeding. In either case, the doctor may order half-strength solution, or change the solution.

But, if your patient complains of nausea or begins to vomit, the tube may have slipped back into her stomach. Stop the feeding, and notify the doctor.

Important: In any event, restart the tube feeding only as ordered by the doctor. Document the procedure in your nurses' notes.

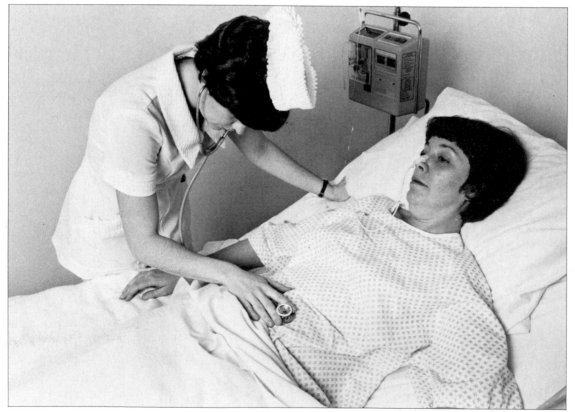

Special problems

Your patient's scheduled for a barium enema, so the doctor has ordered a suppository and nonretention enema to complete the 24-hour preparation.

Do you know why he ordered a nonretention enema instead of a retention one? Or how to prevent your patient from suffering intestinal cramps during these procedures?

Suppose you're caring for a patient who's incontinent? In this case, you'll have to provide good perineal skin care, and help ease your patient's anxieties. Do you know how?

In this section, you'll learn what to do in these situations. You'll also find out how to:
• care for a patient with a perineal wound.
• prepare a patient for endoscopy.
• identify different types of enemas.

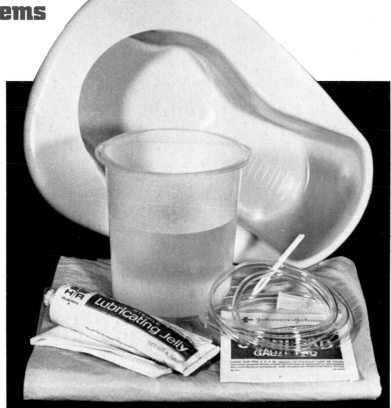

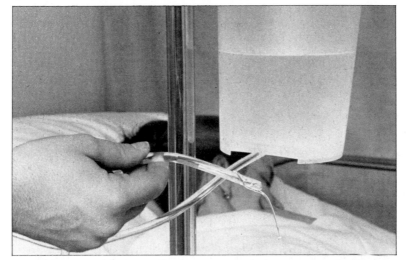

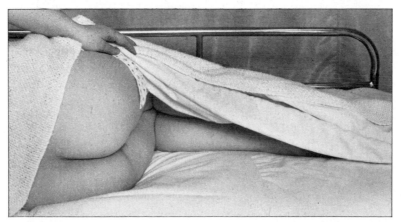

Administering a nonretention enema

1 *Let's say the doctor orders a nonretention enema for your patient. You'll administer it using almost the same procedure as the one described on pages 127 and 128. But, some differences do exist. Read this photostory to find out what they are.*

First, prepare your patient for the procedure. Gather the necessary equipment: enema can, enema solution, tubing, slide clamp, bed-saver pad, water-soluble lubricant, paper towels, 4"x4" gauze pads, and bedpan. You also need an I.V. pole.

Note: You may use an enema bag instead of an enema can and a rectal tube, but both require the clamp.

Explain the procedure to your patient.

2 Heat the enema solution to about 105° F. (40.6° C.) to avoid stimulating peristalsis and to reduce patient discomfort. Test the solution's temperature by using a bath thermometer. Pour the solution into the enema container.

Hang the container on the I.V. pole 12" to 18" (30 to 46 cm) above your patient's bed. Let some solution flow through the tubing to remove any air. Clamp the tubing.

Important: If your female patient has a reproductive system disorder, hang the container level with the upper portion of her hip.

3 Close the door and pull the bed curtain for your patient's privacy. Place your patient on her left side with her right knee flexed (Sims' position). If she's uncomfortable, position her on her right side or back.

Place the bed-saver pad under your patient's left buttock, and tuck part of it between her legs, to catch any fluid that may escape from her rectum. Expose her anus, but provide a drape to keep her warm and avoid embarrassment.

Special problems

Administering a nonretention enema continued

4 Now, place a small amount of lubricant on a paper towel. Lubricate the tip of the rectal tube or catheter by rolling it in the lubricant.

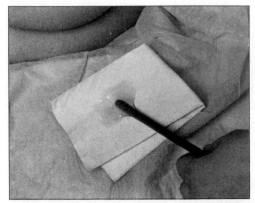

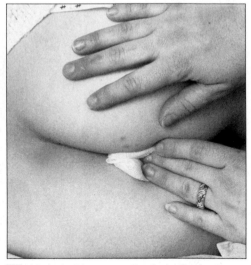

5 Next, tell your patient to breathe deeply as you carefully advance the tube about 4" (10.2 cm) past her internal anal sphincter, directing the tip toward the umbilicus.

Then, open the clamp slightly, allowing the solution to flow gradually into her rectum.

If your patient feels cramps or an urge to defecate, stop the flow by pinching the tube. Ask her to breathe deeply, to help her relax. Then, continue the flow until the container's *almost* empty.

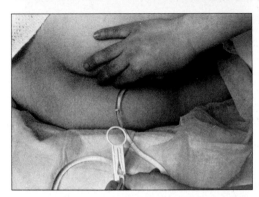

6 Now, clamp the tube. Remove the tubing from your patient's rectum.

Important: Never allow the container to empty before you clamp it, or you may infuse air into the rectum .

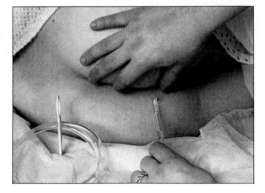

7 Next, hold your patient's buttocks together until her urge to defecate diminishes. Or, press on her anus with a 4"x4" gauze pad. Encourage her to try holding the enema for at least 10 minutes, but keep the bedpan within her reach if she must defecate sooner. When she's ready to expel the enema, assist her onto the bedpan, or help her into the bathroom (if the doctor permits).

If your patient can't expel the enema solution after a reasonable time period, you may have to withdraw it for her, as described on page 130.

Now, wash and dry your patient's buttocks. Ventilate her room or use an air freshener, if necessary.

Then, document the procedure, noting the following: type and quantity of enema solution used; amount, color, and consistency of feces expelled; amount of expelled flatus; any reduction in abdominal distention; and your patient's tolerance for the procedure.

PATIENT PREPARATION

Preparing the patient for a medicated retention enema

Has the doctor ordered a medicated retention enema for your patient? If so, you'll need to properly prepare your patient. Begin by checking your patient's condition. If he's constipated, the feces may block the enema and interfere with drug absorption. Does he have diarrhea? This may cause the drug to be expelled before it's absorbed. An inflamed rectum may be exacerbated by an enema. Notify the doctor if any of these conditions exist.

In addition, follow these guidelines:
• Schedule the procedure before meals. A full stomach

may stimulate peristalis, making retention difficult.
• Explain to your patient what the procedure is and why it's necessary. Stress the importance of retaining the enema for the prescribed time so the medication is fully absorbed.
• Make sure the solution's warmed to the proper temperature before administering. See chart on pages 130 and 131 for guidelines.
• Finally, make sure your patient empties his bladder and rectum before the procedure, reducing peristalsis.

Administering a retention enema

1 *Consider this situation: You're going to give a retention enema to 45-year-old Judy Mason. But before you do, prepare your patient for the enema, as explained on page 126.*

Then, gather the equipment you'll need: a pitcher or small container to hold the enema solution, a bulb syringe with bulb removed, a rectal tube or enema tubing, water-soluble lubricant, a bed-saver pad, a paper towel, 4"x4" gauze pads, a bedpan, and a hemostat.

Or, use one of the prepackaged enemas, such as Fleet®.

Heat the enema solution to about 105° F. (40.6° C.). To check the solution's temperature, use a bath thermometer, or pour a small amount over the inside of your wrist.

As you know, by warming the solution prior to administration, you can avoid stimulating peristalsis.

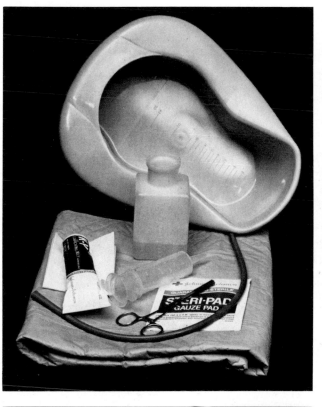

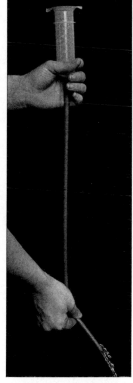

2 To ensure your patient's privacy during this procedure, close the door and adjust her bed curtain. Place Ms. Mason in a left side-lying position with her right knee flexed (Sims' position). This allows the enema solution to flow naturally into the descending colon.

Note: If your patient's uncomfortable in this position, place her on her back or right side instead.

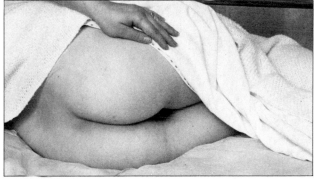

3 Next, place a bed-saver pad under your patient's left buttock. Tuck part of the pad between her legs, as the nurse is doing here.

Expose your patient's anus, but drape the other areas of her body to keep her warm and protect her privacy. Make certain she understands the procedure and reassure her.

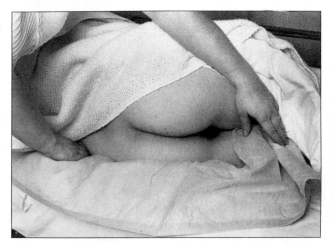

4 Remove the bulb from the syringe and attach the syringe to the rectal tube. Hold the open end of the rectal tube higher than the junction of the syringe and tube, as shown here. Pour a small amount of the solution into the syringe.

Lower the open end of the tube and flush out the air by allowing some solution to flow out. Then, pinch the tube between your fingers, or clamp it.

5 Hold up the open end of the tube and clamp it, as shown in this photo. Keep the syringe attached.

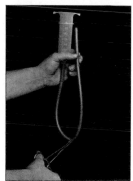

6 Next, squeeze a little water-soluble lubricant onto a paper towel. Roll the tip of the tube in the lubricant, as the nurse is doing here.

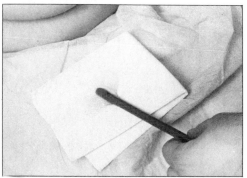

Special problems

Administering a retention enema continued

7 Separate your patient's buttocks so you can see her anus. Ask her to breathe deeply through her mouth as you insert the tube in her anus. Direct the tip of the tube toward Ms. Mason's umbilicus as you advance it about 4" (10.2 cm) past the internal anal sphincter.

Suppose you meet resistance as you advance the tube. Stop immediately. Withdraw the tube slightly and attempt to reinsert it. If you continue to meet resistance, withdraw the tube completely and notify the doctor.

Important: Never force the tube. You may perforate your patient's rectum.

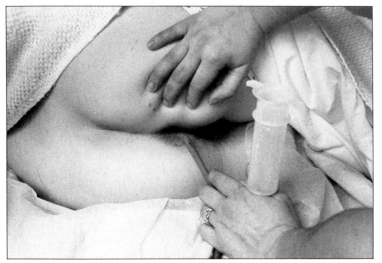

8 Hold the syringe about 5" (12.7 cm) above your patient's anus. Slowly pour the warm solution into the syringe.

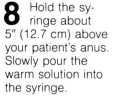

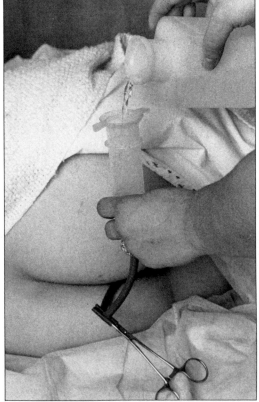

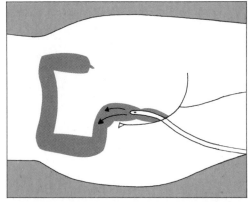

9 Now, remove the clamp, allowing the solution to flow into your patient's anal canal. Don't try to rush the procedure by pouring the solution faster or raising the syringe height. Either of these will increase the fluid pressure in the rectum, stimulating an urge to defecate.

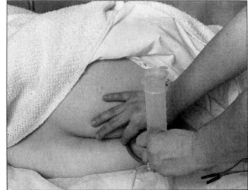

10 What if your patient feels cramps or an urge to defecate? Pinch or clamp the tube and ask her to breathe deeply. When she's relaxed, proceed slowly.

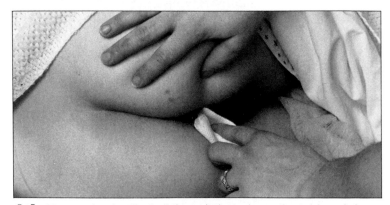

11 After you've instilled all the solution, clamp the tubing. Ask your patient to take a deep breath, and withdraw the tube quickly.

Does your patient have an urge to defecate? Hold her buttocks together until the urge passes. Or, press firmly on her anus with the 4"x4" gauze pad. Then, wash and dry her buttocks. Also, remember to wash your hands.

Ms. Mason should retain the enema for at least 30 minutes. However, the time will vary according to the medication. During this time, try to keep your patient as comfortable and quiet as possible. Leave the bed-saver pad in place and keep the bedpan within her reach.

When the prescribed length of time has passed, tell your patient she may defecate. Then, document the procedure in your notes.

But if your patient has trouble retaining the enema solution, one of the methods described on page 129 may help her.

How to help your patient retain an enema solution

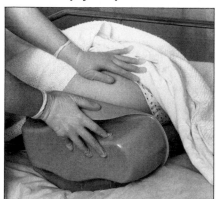

1 *If your patient has difficulty retaining enema solution, follow these guidelines:*

First, put on gloves to protect your hands in case she expels the enema solution suddenly. Protect the bed linen with bed-saver pads. Also, place a bedpan under your patient's left hip and against her left buttock, as shown here.

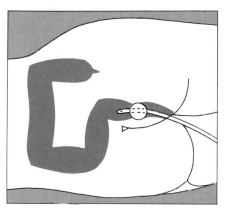

2 To help her retain the enema solution, try using a Foley catheter as a rectal tube (if hospital policy permits). Do this by inserting the catheter as you would a rectal tube. Then, inflate the catheter's balloon with 15 to 20 ml water. Slowly pull the catheter back against your patient's internal anal sphincter. After the catheter's clamped, the balloon will seal off her rectum.

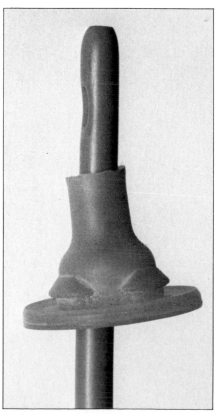

3 Or, try this method to seal off your patient's rectum. Snip off the tip of a baby bottle nipple. Then, slip the nipple over the end of the tube or catheter, as shown in the photo. By pressing the nipple against your patient's anus, you'll help prevent solution from seeping out.

How to withdraw enema solution

1 *If your patient hasn't expelled nonretention enema solution after 30 minutes, you'll have to withdraw it.*

Begin by placing your patient in a right side-lying position. This will allow her descending colon to empty naturally (see inset). Be sure a bed-saver pad is tucked under her buttocks.

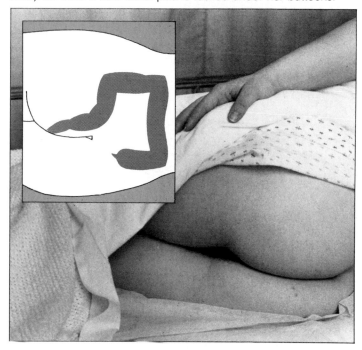

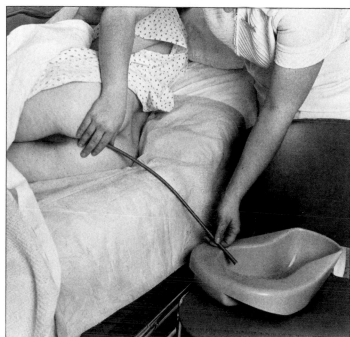

2 Now, place the bedpan on a chair by her bed, below the level of her rectum. Lubricate and insert one end of a tube (size 22 to 30 French) into her rectum, as shown here. Place the other end of the tube in the bedpan, which allows gravity to help withdraw the enema solution.

Special problems

How to withdraw enema solution continued

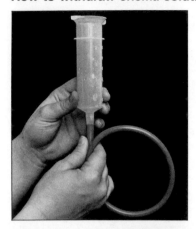

3 Suppose your patient still doesn't expel the solution. Then, you may have to siphon it out. But, first check your hospital's policy. In some hospitals, you'll need a doctor's order before proceeding.

To siphon enema solution, position your patient on her right side, with the bed-saver pad under her buttocks. Remove the bulb from a bulb syringe and attach the syringe to the rectal tube (see photo).

Note: You can substitute a small funnel for the syringe.

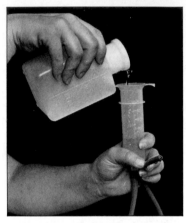

4 Hold the end of the tube upward. Pour warm tap water into the syringe so it's half filled. Then, flush air from the tube and clamp it.

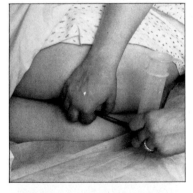

5 Now, apply water-soluble lubricant to the end of the tube and insert it into your patient's rectum about 4" (10 cm). Make sure you hold the syringe above her anus. Next, unclamp the tube, allowing a small amount of water to flow into your patient.

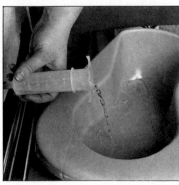

6 Next, invert the syringe over the bedpan. Pressure and gravity will help drain the solution from your patient's rectum.

Document the procedure in your nurses' notes. Be sure to describe the amount, color, and consistency of the siphoned solution and any expelled feces.

Nurses' guide to enemas

You're probably familiar with many different types of retention and nonretention enemas. As you know, a retention enema is usually medicated and retained from 10 to 30 minutes. A nonretention enema is given for constipation and expelled after 10 minutes.

But no matter which type of enema you're administering, always provide for your patient's privacy. Then, place him in a left side-lying position (if possible), and reassure him.

To compare and learn about the different types of enemas and the necessary nursing procedures, read this chart.

Important: When administering an enema to a patient with a history of cardiac problems, always observe him carefully. The enema may stimulate a vagal response, causing cardiac arrhythmia.

TYPE OF ENEMA

Soapsuds
Nonretention

Oil
Retention

Dioctyl sodium sulfosuccinate (Colace)
Retention

Kayexalate* in sorbitol
Retention

Quassia
Retention

Neomycin sulfate
Retention

Milk and molasses
Retention

*Available in both the United States and in Canada

SOLUTION	PURPOSE	NURSING CONSIDERATIONS
• Usually a prepackaged, pH-neutral soap (such as castile) mixed in 1,000 ml water	• Cleans colon and rectum of impacted feces. • Removes coated barium (used in diagnostic tests) from rectum and colon.	• Hang enema administration set no higher than 18″ (46 cm) above the patient's rectum. • Before beginning the procedure, expel all air from tubing. • Warm enema solution to 105° F. (40.6° C.). • Carefully insert lubricated tube about 4″ (10.2 cm) into patient's anus. Do not force it. • If patient develops cramps, stop solution flow. Then, after the cramps have subsided, lower administration set to decrease the flow. • Instill as much solution as patient can retain.
• Prepackaged mineral oil (150 to 175 ml)	• Softens fecal material to ease evacuation.	• Warm solution to 105° F. (40.6 ° C.) before administering. • Tell patient to retain enema solution for at least 30 minutes, if possible.
• Strength and amount of solution vary, as ordered by doctor.	• Softens and lubricates impacted fecal material.	• Warm solution to 98° F. (36.7 ° C.) before administering.
• Strength and amount of Kayexalate and sorbitol vary, as ordered by doctor. Usually 30 to 50 gm Kayexalate in 150 to 200 ml sorbitol.	• Lowers serum potassium level by promoting fecal excretion of potassium.	• Mix solution thoroughly before administering. • Warm solution to 98° F. (36.7° C.) before administering. • Use small-lumen tube to help reduce rectal irritation and the urge to defecate. • Tell patient to retain solution for 30 minutes. Then, drain solution through rectal tube to remove. • If hospital policy permits, use a Foley catheter with a 30 cc balloon as a rectal tube to help patient retain enema solution. Fill balloon with 15 to 20 ml water. If enema solution leaks, add water up to balloon capacity. • Monitor patient's serum potassium level to evaluate results.
• A mixture of 15 gm Quassia in 600 ml water	• Destroys threadworms, seatworms, and other types of pinworms.	• Administer a cleansing soapsuds enema first, to allow direct contact between Quassia and intestinal lining. • Then administer 250 ml Quassia solution per treatment. • Tell patient to retain solution for 15 to 30 minutes. If hospital policy permits, use Foley catheter with inflated balloon to help patient retain enema. • Repeat procedure daily until all worms are destroyed, as determined by stool culture.
• Strength and amount vary, as ordered by doctor; usually 250 ml of a 0.5% solution.	• Prepares bowel for intestinal surgery by reducing bacteria count. • Reduces ammonia level by decreasing intestinal bacteria. Sometimes used as adjunct therapy for hepatic coma.	• Warm solution to 98° F. (36.7° C.) before administering. • Tell patient to retain solution for at least 30 minutes.
• A mixture of 175 to 250 ml each of milk and molasses	• Relieves flatulence by peristaltic stimulation.	• Warm the milk and molasses to 110° F. (43.3° C.) prior to mixing. • Add milk to molasses slowly. Stir well to blend thoroughly. • Be sure to administer solution at 105° F. (40.6° C.).

Special problems

How to insert a rectal suppository

1 *Preparing to administer a rectal suppository? If so, you'll need: a suppository, glove or finger cot, and water-soluble lubricant. Then, wash your hands.*

If a suppository gets warm, it'll stick to its wrapper. So, before unwrapping, hold the suppository under cold running water until it becomes firm (see inset). Or, place it in the medications refrigerator for a few minutes.

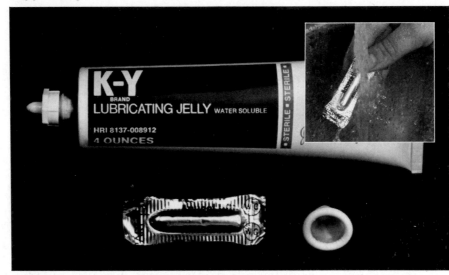

2 Now, provide for your patient's privacy, and explain the procedure to her. Have her lie on either side, whichever she finds most comfortable. Drape her body, leaving only her anus exposed.

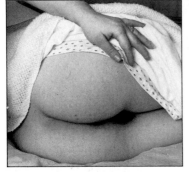

3 Put on a glove or finger cot. Then, take the suppository from the wrapper. Apply water-soluble lubricant to the suppository's tapered end.

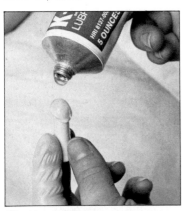

4 Now, separate your patient's buttocks with your ungloved hand, so you can see her anus.

Ask her to take a deep breath. Using your gloved hand, carefully insert the tapered end of the suppository into her rectum. With your forefinger, direct the suppository along her rectal wall toward the umbilicus. Advance it 3" (7.5 cm), or approximately the length of your finger. Be sure the suppository has passed your patient's internal anal sphincter (see inset), or it may be expelled.

Note: Be careful not to push the suppository into a fecal mass.

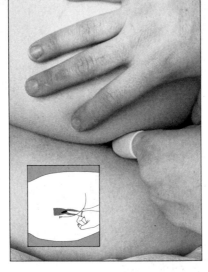

5 After the suppository's in place, remove your finger and take off the glove or finger cot.

Hold your patient's buttocks together or press a 4"x4" gauze pad or tissues against her anus to help suppress any urge to defecate.

Then, use a gauze pad to clean any excess lubricant from her anus. Tell your patient to hold in the suppository for at least 20 minutes.

Now, wash your hands and document the insertion procedure in your nurses' notes.

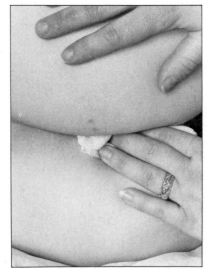

Your role in lower GI endoscopy

Lower gastrointestinal endoscopy allows the doctor to: view rectal and intestinal mucosa; obtain biopsy specimens of suspected pathology; take brushings for cytology; and perform some surgical techniques, such as polyp removal and ligation of internal hemorrhoids.

To prepare your patient for this procedure:

• give clear liquids for 24 to 48 hours prior to the exam, if it's colonoscopy. No diet restrictions are necessary for a patient undergoing sigmoidoscopy or proctoscopy. Be sure to stress to your patient the importance of any diet restriction.

• be ready to administer laxatives, suppositories, or enemas, as ordered, to help evacuate your patient's bowels. If he's an outpatient, you'll have to instruct him on the administration of a laxative and giving enemas.

• explain the examination to him. Be sure to tell him it will be uncomfortable, but probably not painful.

• administer a sedative or pain medication, as ordered.

• help him into Sims' or a knee-chest position for the exam.

When the doctor begins inserting the tube, be prepared to assist, as needed. Monitor your patient's vital signs, and continue to reassure him. In addition, any specimens should be labeled with the patient's name, his hospital identification number, time and date. Then, send the specimens to the lab for analysis. Document everything in your nurses' notes.

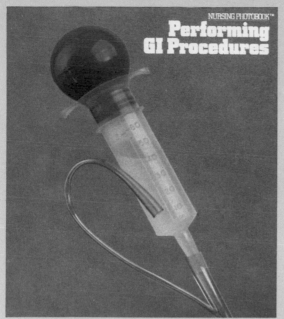

NURSING PHOTOBOOK™
Performing GI Procedures

Now you can update your GI nursing skills with this important new PHOTOBOOK, *Performing GI Procedures*. Clear photographs and concise captions show you step by step how to cope with all types of GI disorders. You'll find complete information on selecting, applying, and removing ostomy pouches, skin barriers, and adhesives. And here's all you need to know to:

- Perform an iced gastric lavage
- Care for a patient with hepatitis
- Drain a continent ileostomy
- Use a volumetric pump to administer a tube feeding
- And much, much more.

Examine this PHOTOBOOK...new from *Nursing82*...for 10 days, free! Send in your order card today.

This is your order card. Send no money.

☐ **YES.** I want to subscribe to the series. Please send me *Performing GI Procedures* as my first volume. If I decide to keep it, I will pay $12.95, plus shipping and handling. I understand that I will receive an exciting new PHOTOBOOK approximately every other month on the same 10-day, free-examination basis. There is no minimum number of books I must buy, and I may cancel my subscription any time.

109-PB

☐ I don't want the series. Just send me *Performing GI Procedures*. I will pay $13.95, plus shipping and handling for each copy.
Please send me _____ copies and bill me. 1PP-09

Name _____

Address _____

City _____

State _____ Zip Code _____

Offer valid in U.S. only   Price is subject to change

10-DAY FREE TRIAL

USE THE CARD ABOVE TO:

1. **Subscribe to the NURSING PHOTOBOOK™ series (and save $1.00 on each book you buy)**

or

2. **Buy *Performing GI Procedures* without joining the series (and pay only $13.95 for each copy)**

© 1982 Intermed Communications, Inc.

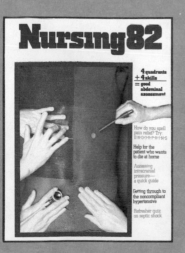

Nursing82

GET ACQUAINTED WITH THE WORLD'S LARGEST NURSING JOURNAL TODAY!

Mail the postage-paid card at right. ▶

Keep your nursing skills growing...with *Nursing82*.

Keep up to date on the latest breakthroughs in nursing care every month in *Nursing82*. With *Nursing82*, you'll be the first to learn about the new techniques and procedures that will mean more skills and knowledge for you... better care for your patients. All in a magazine that's easy to read, easy to understand, and colorfully illustrated to show *you* how to improve your nursing care.

☐ Send me 1 year (12 issues) of *Nursing82*. My check for $16 is enclosed, saving me $4 off the regular $20 price.

☐ Please bill me later for $16.

Name _____

Address _____

City _____ State _____ Zip _____

I am an: ☐ RN ☐ LPN ☐ Other   Do you work in a hospital? ☐ Yes ☐ No

7P09

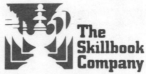

Introduce yourself to the brand-new NURSING PHOTOBOOK™ series

…the remarkable breakthrough in nursing education that can change your career. Each book in this unique series contains detailed *Photostories*… and tables, charts, and graphs to help you learn important new procedures. And each handsome PHOTOBOOK offers you • 160 illustrated, fact-filled pages • brilliant, high-contrast photographs • convenient 9"x10½" size • durable, hardcover binding • carefully chosen bibliography • complete index. Watch the experts at work showing you how to… administer drugs… teach your patient about his illness and its treatment… minimize trauma… understand doctors' diagnoses… increase patient comfort… and much more. Discover how you can become a better nurse by joining this exciting new series. You can examine each PHOTOBOOK at your leisure… for 10 days *absolutely free!*

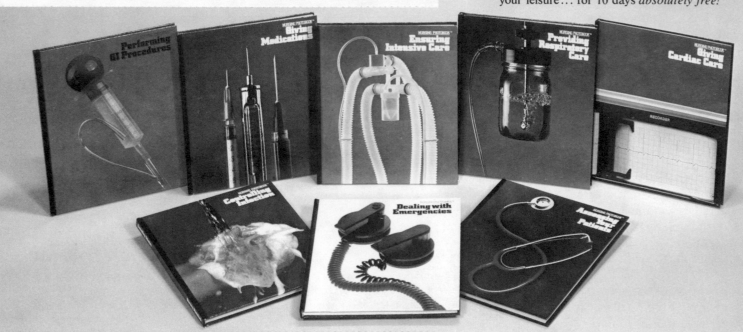

Be sure to mail the postage-paid card at left to reserve *your* first copy of *Nursing82.*

Nursing82 gives you clear, concise instruction in "hands-on" nursing. Every issue brings you in-depth clinical articles about the newest developments in nursing care—what's being discovered, researched, treated, cured. You'll learn about the new procedures, new techniques, new medications, and new equipment that will mean more skills and knowledge for you…better care for your patients!

Order your subscription today!

Care guidelines for the patient with a perineal wound

Consider the patient with a perineal wound. To promote healing and reduce the risk of skin breakdown, perform each of these procedures routinely:
• Observe the perineal area for signs of skin breakdown. Also check for redness, drainage, or open sutures. Document all observations in your nurses' notes.
• Clean the wound several times a day with cleansing solution or disinfectant, as ordered by the doctor. If your patient has a rectal catheter in place, also keep the catheter and catheter site clean and free of dried blood and feces.
• Irrigate the wound every 6 to 12 hours with a solution of half hydrogen peroxide and half sterile water (or other solution), as ordered.
• Give patient a sitz bath at least twice daily, as ordered, to soothe rectal irritation.
• After each sitz bath, direct a heat lamp at the perineal area for 15 minutes, as ordered, to promote drying and healing.
• Administer pain medication, as ordered.
• During the healing process, expect to see some tissue sloughing. But, notify the doctor if you see any of the following complications: excessive drainage, inflammation, or infection.

Preparing your patient for a barium enema

The doctor will order a barium enema for your patient to help detect possible polyps, tumors, and lesions in the colon. A barium enema takes about 15 minutes and is uncomfortable—but not painful—to the patient.

How does a barium enema work? First, the doctor or X-ray technician administers barium into the rectum through a balloon-tipped catheter. The barium outlines your patient's lower GI tract so X-rays can be taken—and eventually evaluated by the doctor.

Before the procedure
What role do you play in this procedure? Your first job is to prepare your patient properly. First, at least 24 hours before the test, thoroughly explain the procedure and its purpose to your patient.

Then, follow these guidelines, as ordered by the doctor:
• Place your patient on a clear liquid diet 24 hours before the procedure.
• Hang a sign above your patient's bed indicating his temporary diet restriction. Instruct visitors and hospital personnel to check at the nurses' station before giving your patient food or fluids.
• Administer laxatives, as well as an enema, to cleanse your patient's colon. If your patient has inflammatory bowel disease, use only a gentle cleansing enema.

After the procedure
In most cases, about 2 hours after the procedure, give your patient 1 ounce each of milk of magnesia and mineral oil. In the evening, administer a 1-liter normal saline solution enema, followed by a second saline solution enema the next morning. This prevents the barium from hardening in your patient's colon, causing an obstruction. In addition, encourage your patient to drink plenty of water. Be sure to warn your patient that his stool will appear white until all barium's expelled.

Document all preparations in your notes.

The chart below outlines steps for 24-, 18-, and 12-hour barium-enema preparation regimens when using the Fleet® prep kit. Study it carefully.

24-HOUR PREP

DAY BEFORE EXAM

• **8 a.m.** Have patient eat light meal
• **9 a.m.** Have patient drink 8 oz. clear liquid
• **10 a.m.** Have patient drink 8 oz. clear liquid
• **11 a.m.** Have patient drink 8 oz. clear liquid
• **12:30 p.m.** (or ½ hour before meal) Have patient drink a mixture of 1½ oz. Fleet Phospo®-Soda and one-half glass of cool water. Then, have him immediately drink 8 oz. of water.
   Provide your patient with a clear liquid meal. Don't give him solid foods or dairy products.
• **2 p.m.** Have patient drink 8 oz. clear liquid
• **3 p.m.** Have patient drink 8 oz. clear liquid
• **4 p.m.** Have patient drink 8 oz. clear liquid
• **6 p.m.** Provide patient with light liquid meal. Don't give him solid foods or dairy products.
• After eating, have patient swallow four yellow Fleet bisacodyl tablets whole with a glass of water.

DAY OF EXAM
• Don't give patient breakfast

1 hour before
• Administer a Fleet bisacodyl enema.

18-HOUR PREP

DAY BEFORE EXAM

• **12 Noon** Have patient eat light meal
• **2 p.m.** Have patient drink 8 oz. clear liquid
• **3 p.m.** Have patient drink 8 oz. clear liquid
• **4 p.m.** Have patient drink 8 oz. clear liquid
• **6 p.m.** (or 1½ hour before meal) Have patient drink a mixture of 1½ oz. Fleet Phospho-Soda and one-half glass of cool water. Then, instruct patient to immediately drink 8 oz. of water.
   Provide patient with clear liquid meal. Don't give him solid foods or dairy products.
• **8 p.m.** Have patient drink 8 oz. clear liquid
• **9 p.m.** Have patient drink 8 oz. clear liquid
• Between 9 p.m. and 10 p.m. Have patient swallow four yellow Fleet bisacodyl tablets whole with 8 oz. of water

DAY OF EXAM
• 8 a.m. Provide patient with a clear liquid meal. Don't give patient solid foods or dairy products.
• 9 a.m. Have patient drink three 8 oz. glasses of water prior to reporting for his exam

1 hour before
• Administer a Fleet bisacodyl enema.

12-HOUR PREP

DAY BEFORE EXAM

• **12 Noon** Have patient eat light meal
• **2 p.m.** Have patient drink 8 oz. clear liquid
• **3 p.m.** Have patient drink 8 oz. clear liquid
• **4 p.m.** Have patient drink 8 oz. clear liquid
• **6 p.m.** (or ½ hour before meal) Have patient drink mixture of 1½ oz. Fleet Phospho-Soda and one-half glass of cool water. Then, instruct patient to immediately drink 8 oz. of water.
   Provide patient with a clear liquid meal. Don't give him solid foods or dairy products.
• **7 p.m.** Have patient drink 8 oz. clear liquid
• **8 p.m.** Have patient drink 8 oz. clear liquid
• **9 p.m.** Have patient drink 8 oz. clear liquid
• Between 9 p.m. and 10 p.m. Have patient swallow four yellow Fleet bisacodyl tablets whole with 8 oz. of water.

DAY OF EXAM
• Don't give patient breakfast

1 hour before
• Administer a Fleet bisacodyl enema.

Special problems

Caring for the incontinent patient

1 *If your patient's incontinent, you'll have to know how to provide comfort and emotional support, and care for her skin properly. By doing this, you can help reduce undue embarrassment and prevent skin irritation and breakdown. This photostory will show you how.*

Note: The nurse is using Sween perineal care products and a Procter & Gamble Attends® disposable brief.

Begin by gathering the following equipment: Peri-Wash®, Peri-Care®, Sween Cream™ (or soap, water, and lotion), two washcloths, towel, proper size Attends disposable brief, and gloves (optional).

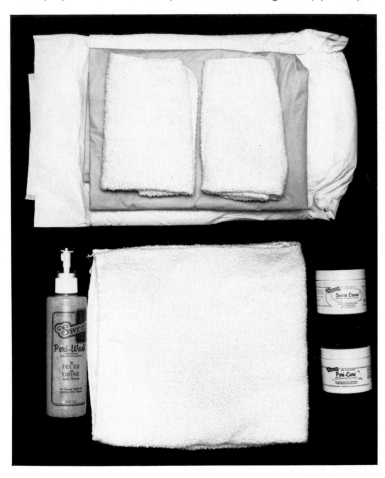

2 Then, provide complete privacy for your patient. Have her lie on her side and remove her used disposable brief. Wrap it in a bed-saver pad and discard it in the utility room—not in your patient's wastebasket. Then, wash your hands thoroughly.

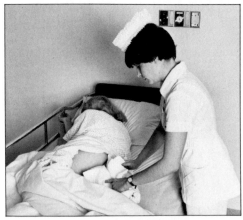

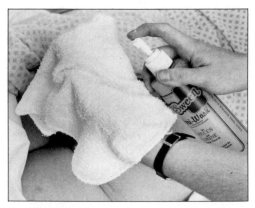

3 Use a water-moistened washcloth sprayed with Peri-Wash to clean your patient's perineum of any feces. Work from the center of the perineum outward.

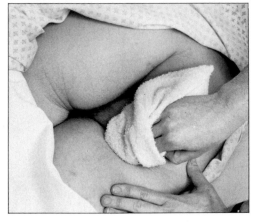

4 Then, using the same technique, rinse the perineum with a clean, water-moistened washcloth.

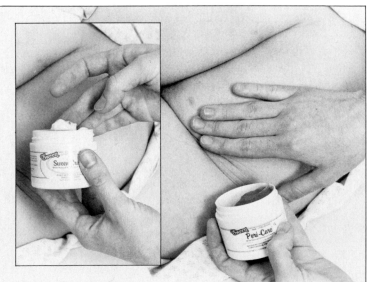

5 Next, pat the area completely dry with a towel. Then, check for signs of skin breakdown. If the skin appears healthy, apply Peri-Care to the area. As you know, gentle massaging helps increase the blood supply to your patient's buttocks and sacral area. But, never massage directly on top of a reddening, irritated area. Instead, massage around it.

[Inset] But, suppose the perineum looks red or irritated. Apply Sween Cream over the perineum; then apply Peri-Care.

6 Now, you're ready to apply the Attends. Place an opened Attends on the bed, with the tapes toward your patient's upper body. Then, fold lengthwise the back flap that's closest to your patient's body. Make sure the waist is aligned with the small of your patient's back.

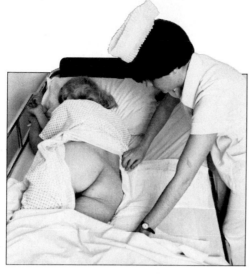

7 Next, roll your patient over the brief and onto her other side. Unfold the back flap.

8 Roll your patient onto her back. She should be positioned evenly on the Attends.
   But if she isn't, roll her away from the side where the largest portion of brief is. Tuck more brief under her and roll her over the brief, onto her other side. Pull the brief out.

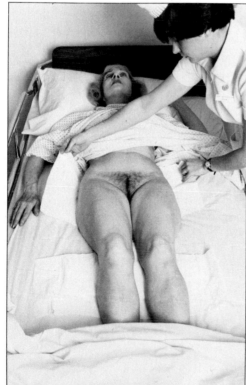

9 Lift the front flap up between her legs. The gathers should fit snugly in her upper leg creases.

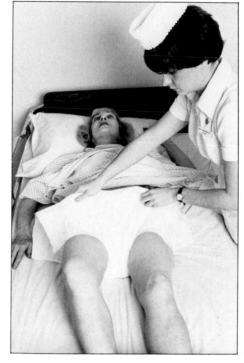

10 Now, peel off the backing from the right leg tape. Gently pull the front and back flaps together in a slightly upward direction. When the area around the tape begins to stretch, fasten the tape to the front flap.
   Important: To ensure a snug fit, angle the tape slightly. Repeat this procedure on the left side.

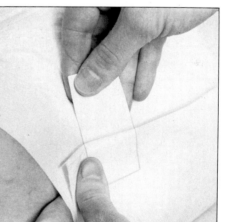

11 Peel the backing from the right waist tape. Pull the front and back flaps together until the area around the tape begins to stretch. Smooth the tape into place.
   Follow the same procedure for attaching the left waist tape.
   Change the Attends whenever it becomes soiled, to maintain your patient's skin integrity and promote her comfort.

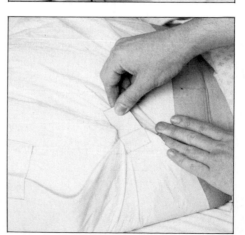

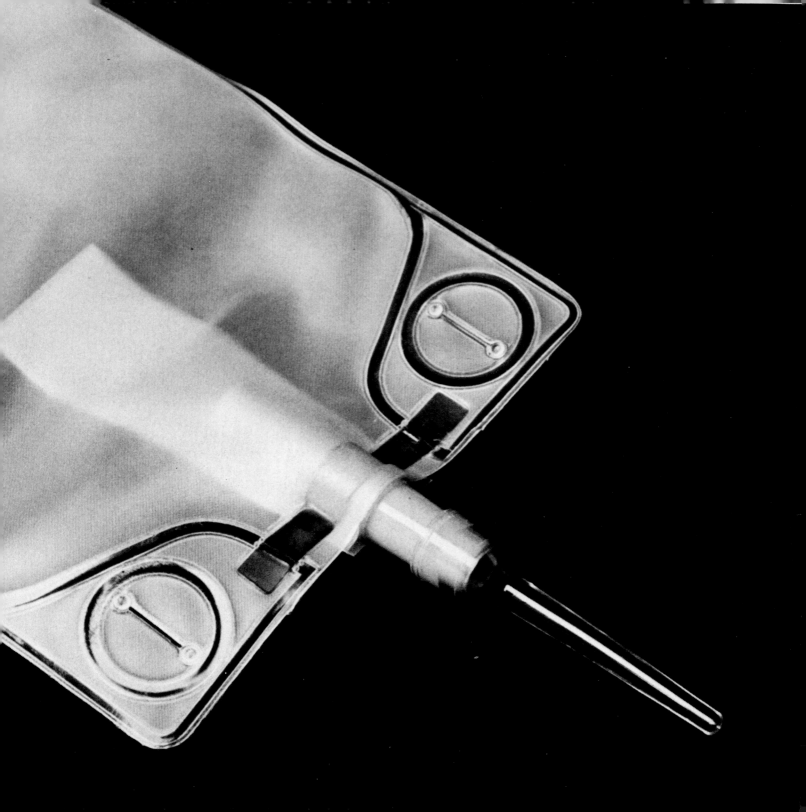

Managing Other Digestive Problems

Gallbladder disorders
Hepatic disorders
Pancreatic disorders

Gallbladder disorders

Caring for a patient with a gallbladder disorder requires special skills. For example, let's say the doctor orders an oral cholecystogram for your patient. Do you know how to prepare your patient properly? When to administer the dye tablets? Or, what to do if your patient goes into anaphylactic shock?

What about caring for the patient who's had a cholecystectomy? Do you know:
• how to reinforce his dressing?
• how to keep his T tube in place?
• how to use Montgomery straps?

If you're unsure about the answers to any of these questions, study the next few pages carefully. You'll find detailed information that'll help you gain a better understanding of gallbladder disorders and their treatment.

PATIENT PREPARATION

Preparing your patient for a cholecystectomy

Is your patient scheduled for a cholecystectomy? If so, he probably is worried about how losing his gallbladder will affect his lifestyle. Take the mystery out of the surgery by anticipating and answering his questions.

Begin by explaining how the gallbladder functions and how his body can gradually adjust to its absence. Bring along an illustration of the GI tract to help with your explanation.

Remember also to tell your patient what to expect after surgery. Be sure to explain the purpose of the I.V. line, Penrose drain, and the nasogastric (NG) and T tubes he'll have in place. Assure him that as his condition improves, all of these will be removed eventually. Explain that his incision will hurt, but remind your patient that the doctor will order pain medication for him. Tell him to request the medication if your patient's in pain.

Before surgery, teach your patient how to prevent respiratory and vascular complications by turning, coughing, deep breathing, and performing leg exercises after surgery. Remind him that these actions will hurt temporarily because of his incision, but assure him that he can have pain medication.

Tell your patient that once he's able to take foods and fluids orally (usually within 2 to 3 days postop), he'll be placed on a low-fat diet. Assure him he'll gradually return to a more normal diet, and be able to eat many foods that caused him discomfort before surgery. Encourage your patient to add new foods to his diet, one at a time. By doing this, he'll determine which foods he can tolerate and which he can't.

How to care for a patient after a cholecystectomy

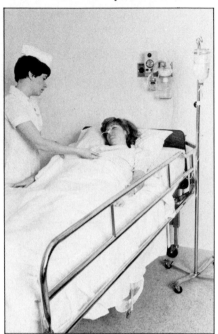

1 It's 3 p.m. and 26-year-old Amy Morrison has been transferred to your unit from the recovery room. Just 2 hours ago, Ms. Morrison had a cholecystectomy because of gallstones. She has a Penrose drain and sutured T tube at her incision site. The T tube is connected to a bile drainage bag, which is held against her abdomen with a rubber belt. In addition, your patient has a clamped nasogastric (NG) tube and an I.V. line in place. To properly care for her, follow these steps.

Begin by reassuring Ms. Morrison. Explain each procedure as you perform it, even if she seems groggy from the anesthesia.

Place her in a low or semi-Fowler's position, whichever is more comfortable for her.

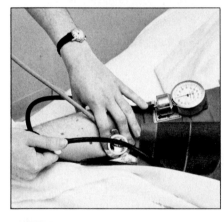

2 Next, take Ms. Morrison's blood pressure, pulse, and respiration rate. Record your findings. Take her vital signs every 2 hours until they stabilize.

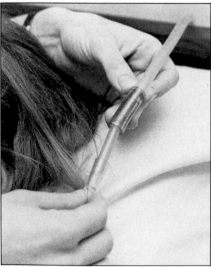

3 Now, unpin your patient's NG tube from her gown. Unclamp the tube and attach it to intermittent low suction, as ordered. The doctor will probably want you to irrigate her NG tube every 2 hours with normal saline solution to ensure patency (see pages 62 and 63 for details).

Note: Be sure to provide good mouth care while Ms. Morrison's NG tube is in place.

4 Closely examine the dressing over Ms. Morrison's incision, noting drainage color. If all's well, the drainage will appear pinkish. Within 48 hours, it'll become straw-colored. But, if the drainage appears bloody (possible internal bleeding), purulent (possible infection), or bile-green (possible suture line separation), notify the doctor.

Nursing tip: Check your patient's bed linens for drainage.

Then, draw a circle around the drainage on your patient's dressing, as shown here. Also, record the time, and initial the dressing. Continue to check Ms. Morrison's dressing every 2 hours during the first 24 hours, and mark the drainage, as described above.

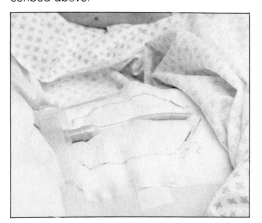

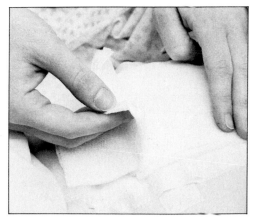

5 In most cases, the doctor makes the first dressing change 24 hours after surgery. But, suppose your patient's dressing becomes saturated before that time. Then, reinforce it by taping additional 4"x4" sterile gauze pads in place, as shown here.

Important: If you have to reinforce the dressing more than twice during the first 6 postop hours, notify the doctor.

Change Ms. Morrison's dressing every 24 hours, or more often if it becomes wet or soiled (see pages 141 to 144 for details).

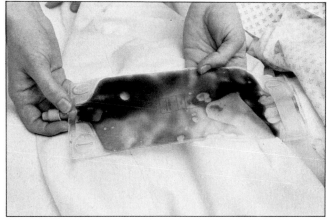

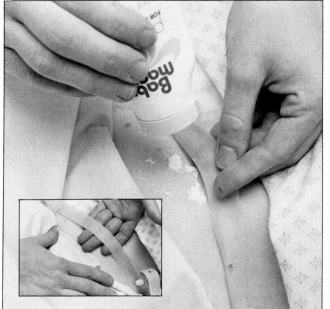

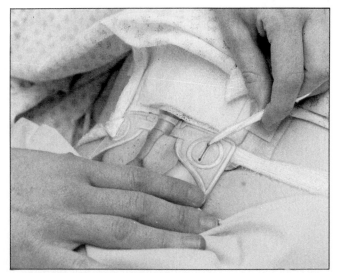

6 Next, note the color and consistency of the drainage in Ms. Morrison's bile bag.

Immediately following surgery, the drainage will appear bloody. After about 6 hours, expect the drainage to look green and viscous. But if it remains bloody, notify the doctor.

Also, check the entire length of your patient's T tube for twisting. If you see any, carefully straighten the tube to prevent blockage.

7 Now, closely examine the skin under the rubber belt. Continue to check Ms. Morrison's skin every 4 hours.

Nursing tip: Apply powder or 4"x4" gauze pads under the belt to help reduce irritation.

[Inset] To check belt tightness, slip your fingers between the belt and Ms. Morrison's skin.

8 If your patient perspires heavily or develops a rash or redness under the rubber belt, try substituting a belt made from umbilical tape or rolled gauze. To do this, slip one end of the gauze strip through the belt opening and knot it. Then, wrap the strip around your patient's waist and attach it to the opposite belt opening.

Gallbladder disorders

How to care for a patient after a cholecystectomy continued

9 When the bile bag is two thirds full (or at least once each shift), empty the bag into a measuring container. Record the amount, color, and consistency of the bile drainage.

If all's well, expect from 300 to 500 ml of bile drainage in the first 24 hours. This amount will decrease gradually to 200 ml or less within 3 to 4 days.

But, what if your patient's bile drainage suddenly decreases to 100 ml within a 24-hour period? Notify the doctor. Ms. Morrison may have a blockage in her common bile duct.

In such a case, the doctor may order a T tube irrigation with normal saline solution. Be ready to assist.

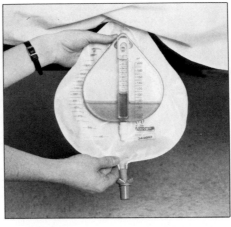

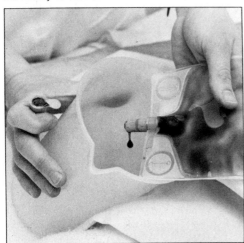

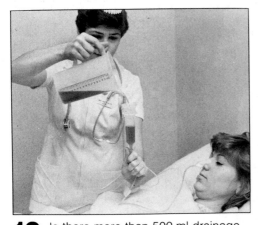

10 Is there more than 500 ml drainage within 24 hours? If so, notify the doctor. Be prepared to administer the bile drainage through your patient's NG tube using a bulb syringe, or orally, as ordered.

🔖 *Nursing tip:* If your patient is to receive the drainage orally, chill and mix the drainage with grape or apple juice. Explain to your patient that the mixture contains medication that will help her digestion.

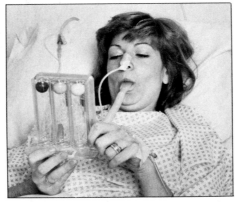

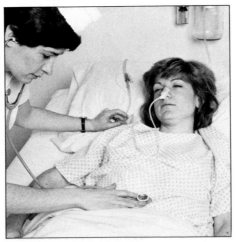

11 Now, observe your patient's urine and stool, noting the color and consistency. Be alert for color changes, such as dark yellow urine (presence of bile), or clay-colored stool (absence of bile in duodenum). If you see either, notify the doctor.

Also, obtain urine and stool specimens for analysis, as ordered. Label each specimen with your patient's name, her hospital ID number, date, and time. Send them to the lab for examination of bile pigment.

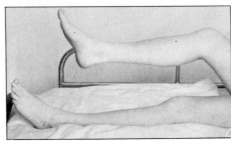

12 To prevent venous stasis, have your patient perform leg exercises, as shown here. Encourage your patient to repeat these exercises every 2 hours, as ordered.

In addition, the doctor may want you to fit your patient with antiembolism (elastic) stockings. For details, see the NURSING PHOTOBOOK *Caring for Surgical Patients.*

13 Now, turn and position your patient and encourage her to deep breathe, cough, and use an incentive spirometer every 2 hours. Be sure to explain that because of her surgery, deep breathing may be painful. However, tell her you'll administer pain medication, when possible, prior to her deep breathing.

14 Auscultate your patient's abdomen daily, listening for bowel sounds, as the nurse is doing here. When the sounds return (about 48 to 72 hours after surgery), notify the doctor. He'll set up a schedule for you to begin clamping your patient's NG tube.

If Ms. Morrison tolerates the clamping procedure, the doctor will probably instruct you to begin giving fluids orally. In your nurses' notes, be sure to record the amount and your patient's tolerance of liquids.

During your patient's recovery, continually monitor her skin and sclera for signs of jaundice, indicating hepatic duct blockage. If you see any signs, notify the doctor.

Document all procedures in your nurses' notes. Remember to include all fluid intake and output records.

Changing a cholecystectomy dressing

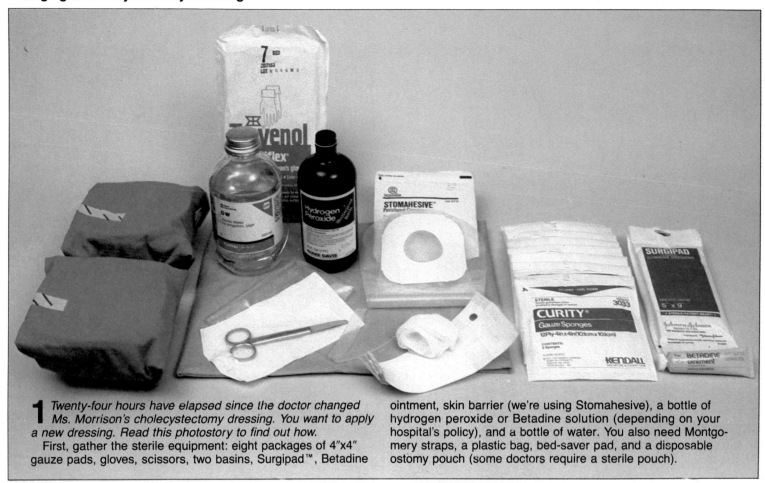

1 *Twenty-four hours have elapsed since the doctor changed Ms. Morrison's cholecystectomy dressing. You want to apply a new dressing. Read this photostory to find out how.*
First, gather the sterile equipment: eight packages of 4"x4" gauze pads, gloves, scissors, two basins, Surgipad™, Betadine ointment, skin barrier (we're using Stomahesive), a bottle of hydrogen peroxide or Betadine solution (depending on your hospital's policy), and a bottle of water. You also need Montgomery straps, a plastic bag, bed-saver pad, and a disposable ostomy pouch (some doctors require a sterile pouch).

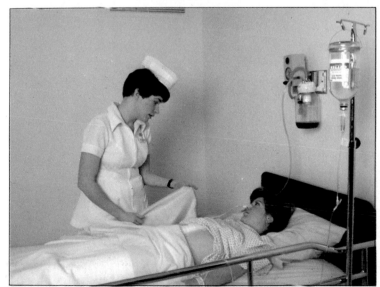

2 Now, explain the procedure to Ms. Morrison. Place her in a supine position. Expose her dressing, but provide a drape to keep her warm.
Place a bed-saver pad under her right side.

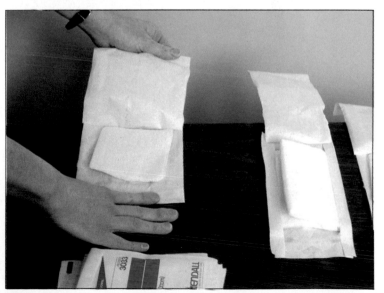

3 Wash your hands thoroughly. Then, maintaining sterility, open the packages of sterile 4"x4" gauze pads. Leaving the pads in their open wrappers, place them on the bedside table. Follow this procedure with the Stomahesive, Surgipad, and scissors.

Gallbladder disorders

Changing a cholecystectomy dressing continued

4 Maintaining sterility, remove the wrappers from both basins, as the nurse is doing here. Place the basins on the bedside table.

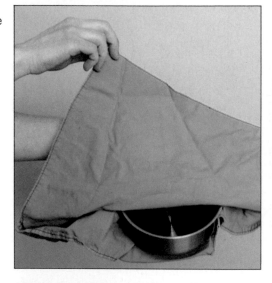

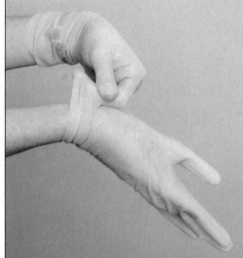

7 Wash your hands again and put on the sterile gloves. From this point on, you'll be using strict aseptic technique.
  Carefully inspect your patient's incision for any discharge or redness. If you see any, notify the doctor.

5 Pour approximately 50 ml of hydrogen peroxide solution into one basin. Then, pour 50 ml sterile water into the other basin.
  Next, place the opened plastic bag on the bed next to your patient.

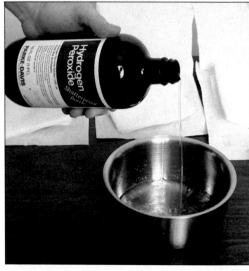

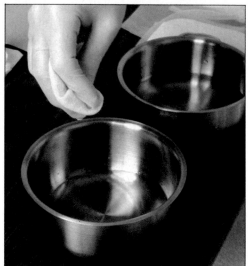

8 Now, dip a 4"x4" gauze pad in the hydrogen peroxide solution. Starting at the incision, gently wipe outward in one motion.
  Then, discard the gauze pad in the plastic bag. Repeat this procedure until you've cleaned the entire incision, using a clean gauze pad with each wiping motion. Be sure to clean around the T tube and Penrose drain.

6 Now, gently remove the old dressing. Be careful not to dislodge Ms. Morrison's T tube or Penrose drain.
  Fold the soiled sides of the dressing together so they don't contaminate your hands.
  Place the dressing in the plastic bag.

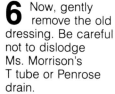

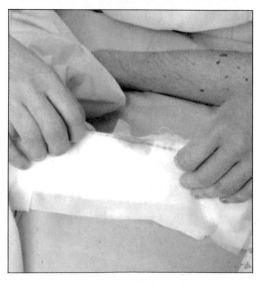

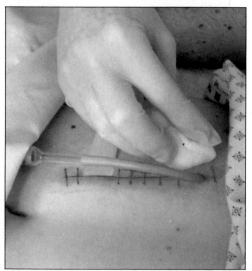

9 Next, rinse the incision site with sterile water, using the technique described above.
  Using 4"x4" gauze pads, pat the area dry. Discard all used gauze pads in the plastic bag.

10 Now, hold two 4"x4" gauze pads together and slit them halfway through the middle. Place these gauze pads on their wrappers.

Note: If you wish, you can use precut drain sponges instead of 4"x4" gauze pads for this part of the procedure.

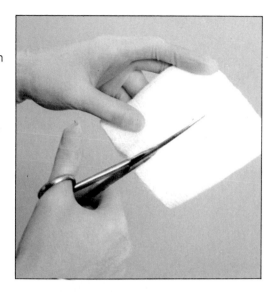

11 Now, using your right hand, remove the cap from the Betadine ointment (or ask your coworker to do this for you). But remember, this hand is no longer sterile.

Using the same hand, squeeze a small amount of ointment onto a 4"x4" gauze pad and discard the gauze pad. This ensures ointment sterility.

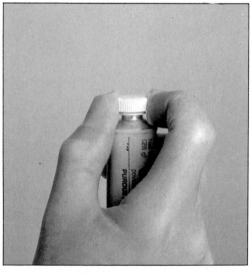

12 Squeeze ointment over Ms. Morrison's entire incision, as shown here. Be careful not to touch her incision with the tip of the ointment tube. Remember, this tube should be used only for Ms. Morrison.

Recap the ointment tube and put it aside.

Note: Some doctors may order an antibiotic ointment other than Betadine.

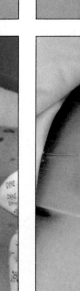

13 In the center of the Stomahesive sheet, cut an opening the size of the Penrose drain, as shown here. Then, remove the Stomahesive's backing.

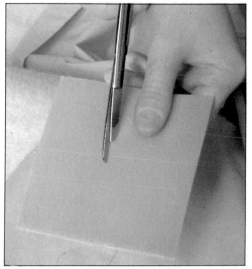

14 Fit the Stomahesive over the Penrose drain. Press firmly, making sure the Stomahesive sticks to your patient's skin.

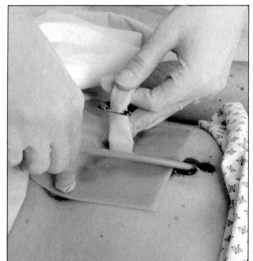

15 Using your left (sterile) hand, take the two slit 4"x4" gauze pads from their wrappers.

Important: Touch only the tops of the pads. Fit them snugly around Ms. Morrison's T tube so the slits overlap, as shown.

Remove your gloves and place them in the plastic bag.

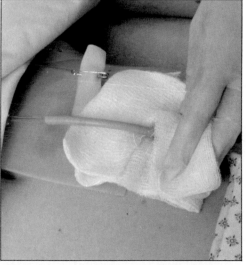

Gallbladder disorders

Changing a cholecystectomy dressing continued

16 Remove the adhesive backing from the faceplate and slip the ostomy pouch over the Penrose drain. Press firmly against the Stomahesive.

Secure the pouch's end with a plastic clamp.

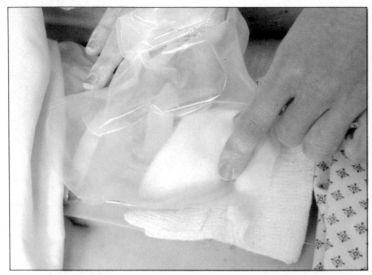

17 Being careful to touch only the top of the Surgipad, place it directly on top of the gauze pads.

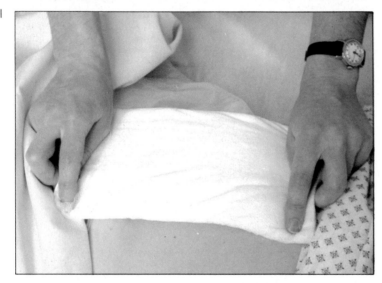

18 Apply Montgomery straps near both ends of the dressing, as the nurse is doing here. Tie each pair of straps together to secure the dressing.

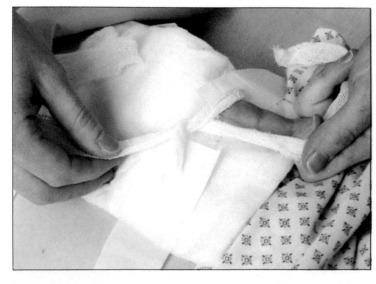

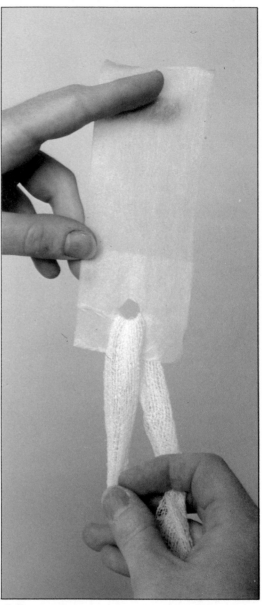

19 Suppose you don't have Montgomery straps. Then, make your own by cutting four 6" (15.2 cm) strips of 2" wide adhesive tape. Fold 2" (5 cm) of the tape back on itself, sticky sides together. Cut a small hole near the edge of the folded end. Place these adhesive strips on either side of the dressing, as described for Montgomery straps.

Then, insert a 12" (30 cm) piece of gauze or umbilical tape through the holes of the facing strips. Tie them together.

Finally, remove the plastic bag from Ms. Morrison's bed and discard it in the utility room. Empty and clean the basins. Return them to the central supply room.

Document the procedure in your nurses' notes.

Clamping the T tube: Your role

Before the doctor removes Ms. Morrison's T tube, he'll instruct you to clamp her tube on an intermittent basis. Here's how:

Explain to Ms. Morrison that you'll clamp her T tube 1 hour before each meal and then unclamp it 1 hour after the meal. Tell her this will aid her digestion by allowing bile to drain directly from the liver into her duodenum.

While the tube's clamped, watch for bile leakage around the base of the T tube. If you see any drainage, or if Ms. Morrison complains of abdominal discomfort, unclamp the tube and notify the doctor. She still may have a blocked common bile duct. In this case, the doctor may want to perform a T tube irrigation with normal saline solution. Be prepared to assist.

If your patient appears to tolerate the clamping procedure, the doctor will probably order a T tube cholangiogram. This special X-ray determines if the common bile duct's patent. Prepare your patient for the test, as described on pages 146 and 147.

If the test result confirms common bile duct patency, the doctor will remove the T tube. Be ready to assist.

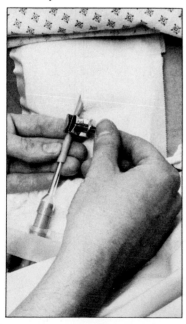

Identifying common gallbladder disorders

How familiar are you with gallbladder disorders? Do you know what signs and symptoms to look for? Or, how to care for your patient properly? The following information acquaints you with four of the most common gallbladder disorders. Study it carefully.

In addition, follow these guidelines when caring for a patient with any type of gallbladder disorder:
* Draw blood to determine electrolyte balance, prothrombin time, complete blood count (CBC), and total bilirubin, as ordered. Label and send specimens to the lab for analysis.
* Administer pain medications, such as meperidine hydrochloride (Demerol*), pentazocine (Talwin*), or morphine, as ordered. If you're administering Demerol or morphine, the doctor may also order nitroglycerin to relieve gallbladder sphincter spasms.
* Obtain urine and stool samples to test for occult blood caused possibly by hypoprothrombinemia.
* Be alert for bleeding from your patient's skin and mucous membranes. If you see any bleeding, notify the doctor. Be prepared to administer vitamin K as ordered.
* Watch for signs of jaundice: yellow sclera or skin; dark yellow urine; and clay-colored stool. If you see any of these signs, notify the doctor.

Acute cholecystitis

Signs and symptoms
* Belching, feeling of fullness, and possible nausea and vomiting after ingesting fatty food
* Moderate to constant pain in right upper quadrant or epigastric area. Possibly referred to right scapula.
* On palpation, tenderness in right upper quadrant, muscle guarding and inability to take deep breath (Murphy's sign)
* Low-grade fever with possible chills
* Leukocyte count between 10,000 and 15,000 per cu mm
* Possible jaundice
* Dehydration, resulting from vomiting and diarrhea

Intervention
* Keep your patient on complete bed rest until acute symptoms (pain, temperature elevation, and dehydration) subside.
* Monitor vital signs every 2 hours until they stabilize and acute symptoms subside.
* Don't give food or fluids until nausea and vomiting have stopped, as ordered.
* Be prepared to insert a nasogastric tube, as ordered.
* Administer I.V. fluids, as ordered, to correct fluid and electrolyte imbalance resulting from dehydration.
* Administer antispasmodics, such as atropine sulfate, papaverine hydrochloride (Cerespan), and propantheline bromide (Pro-Banthine*), I.V., as ordered, to reduce sphincter spasm and control pain.
* Each shift, assess patient's abdomen for increased rigidity, tenderness, or presence of a mass, which may indicate a possible rupture of the gallbladder with peritonitis. Notify the doctor if you see these signs.
* Prepare the patient for cholecystectomy, if ordered by the doctor.

Chronic cholecystitis

Signs and symptoms
* Belching, feeling of fullness, and possible nausea and vomiting after ingesting fatty food
* Mild to moderate right upper quadrant pain that radiates to the back below the right scapular tip
* Low-grade fever
* Constipation
* Leukocyte count between 10,000 and 15,000 per cu mm
* Possible jaundice

Intervention
* Provide low-fat diet. Don't give patient fried foods, butter, margarine, whole milk, or nuts.
* Administer antispasmodics, such as atropine sulfate, papaverine hydrochloride (Cerespan), and propantheline bromide (Pro-Banthine*), I.V., as ordered, to reduce sphincter spasm and control pain.
* Prepare patient for cholecystectomy, if ordered.

Cholelithiasis (gallstones)

Signs and symptoms
* Dyspepsia, flatulence, abdominal discomfort, feeling of fullness, heartburn, and possible nausea and vomiting (3 to 6 hours after ingesting fatty food)
* Moderate to intense steady pain in right upper quadrant or midepigastric area, possibly radiating to back or right shoulder
* Tachycardia; diaphoresis (possibly confused with myocardial infarction pain)
* Fever accompanied by chills
* Possible jaundice

Intervention
* Administer antispasmodics, such as atropine sulfate, papaverine hydrochloride (Cerespan), and propantheline bromide (Pro-Banthine*), I.V., as ordered, to reduce sphincter spasm and control pain.
* Begin I.V. therapy with 1,000 ml normal saline solution, as ordered.
* Be prepared to insert nasogastric tube, if ordered.
* Administer fat-soluble vitamins (A, D, E, and K) I.M. or orally, as ordered. If provided orally, use bile salts (dehydrocholic acid) to aid in vitamin absorption.
* Prepare patient for cholecystectomy, if ordered by the doctor.

*Available in both the United States and in Canada

Gallbladder disorders

Identifying common gall-bladder disorders continued

Cancer of the gallbladder

Signs and symptoms
Early signs and symptoms
• May have no early symptoms.
• Acute episodes of epigastric and right upper abdominal pain
• On palpation, mass in right subcostal area
• Weight loss
Late signs and symptoms
• Persistent severe epigastric and right upper abdominal pain
• Anorexia with severe weight loss
• Nausea, vomiting
• Diarrhea
• Bleeding from skin and mucous membrane
• Generalized weakness
• Ascites
• Possible jaundice

Intervention
• Place air mattress on bed, and turn and position patient every 2 hours to prevent bed sores. Elevate head of bed to facilitate breathing.
• Administer antiemetics, such as diphenhydramine hydrochloride (Benadryl*) or dimenhydrinate (Dramamine*), orally, to help reduce nausea and vomiting.
• Allow patient to eat whatever he can tolerate.
• Administer vitamin and mineral replacements I.M. or orally, as ordered. If provided orally, use with bile salts (dehydrocholic acid) to aid in absorbing fat-soluble vitamins.
• Insert feeding tube, as ordered, if oral feedings are not tolerated.
• Prepare patient for cholecystectomy, if ordered.

Nurses' guide to gallbladder testing

Has it been a while since you've prepared a patient for diagnostic gallbladder testing? If so, the chart that follows will refresh your memory. But remember, some of these tests require the patient to have a normally functioning liver. So, you'll have to check for signs of liver dysfunction before proceeding with the test. For example, watch the patient for signs of jaundice, and draw blood for bilirubin level and liver function studies. If you see signs of jaundice, or if the total serum bilirubin level measures more than 25 mg/100 ml (normal values: 0.7 mg/ 100 ml), suspect liver dysfunction and notify the doctor.

Remember to explain each testing procedure to your patient in words he can understand.

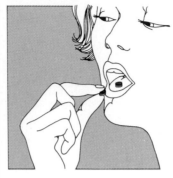

ORAL CHOLECYSTOGRAM

Purpose
• Performed only if patient's liver is functioning normally
• To detect gallstones or duct strictures

Procedure
• Contrast dye is administered orally 12 to 14 hours before X-ray

Nursing preparations
• Obtain accurate history of patient's allergies, especially to iodine and seafood. Remember, the contrast dye used in this test contains iodine.
• Provide patient with a low-fat meal about 16 hours before X-ray.
• Have patient swallow six dye tablets with 8 oz. of water, as ordered, 1 hour after meal.
• Following dye tablet ingestion, notify doctor if patient vomits. The doctor may want you to repeat the dosage, administer a decreased dosage, or order an I.V. cholangiogram instead.
• After dye has been ingested, withhold foods and oral fluids until the X-ray has been completed.
• Closely monitor patient for signs and symptoms of an allergic reaction; for example, rash, diarrhea, and itching. If present, notify the doctor immediately. In rare cases, you may see signs of anaphylactic shock. Be prepared to administer epinephrine hydrochloride (Sus-Phrine*), as ordered. Notify the doctor if these signs appear.

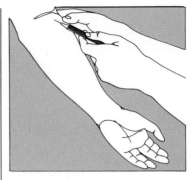

I.V. CHOLANGIOGRAM

Purpose
• Performed postcholecystectomy if symptoms recur
• Performed only if patient's liver is functioning normally

Procedure
• After a test dose of 0.5 ml iodine is administered I.V. (with no adverse reaction in 3 minutes), contrast dye is slowly injected I.V. over a 10 minute period during the X-ray procedure.

Nursing preparations
• Obtain accurate history of patient's allergies, especially to seafood and iodine. Remember the contrast dye used in this test contains iodine.
• Provide patient with a low-fat meal about 16 hours before scheduled X-ray.
• After meal, withhold foods and oral fluids until the X-ray has been completed.
• Warn the patient he may feel a warm, burning sensation when the dye's injected.
• After X-ray procedure, closely monitor patient for signs and symptoms of allergic reaction; for example, rash, diarrhea, and itching. If present, notify the doctor immediately. In rare cases, you may see signs of anaphylactic shock. Be prepared to administer epinephrine hydrochloride (Sus-Phrine*), as ordered. Notify the doctor if these signs appear.

*Available in both the United States and in Canada

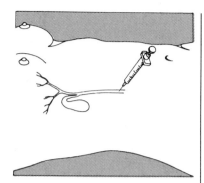

PERCUTANEOUS TRANSHEPATIC
CHOLANGIOGRAM

Purpose
• Patient's liver does not need to be functioning normally to have this test.
• Done prior to cholecystectomy to differentiate between hepatogenic jaundice and obstructive jaundice
• To locate stones in bile ducts
• To detect and diagnose biliary system cancer
• To visualize hepatic ducts, cystic duct, common bile duct, and gallbladder

Procedure
• Contrast dye is injected through abdominal wall into biliary tree, immediately before X-ray.

Nursing preparations
• Obtain accurate history of patient's allergies, especially to seafood and iodine. Remember, the contrast dye used in this test contains iodine.
• Withhold food and oral fluids for 10 to 12 hours before X-ray.
• Administer a sedative 1 hour before X-ray, as ordered.
• After the X-ray procedure, closely monitor patient for signs and symptoms of allergic reaction; for example, rash, diarrhea, and itching. If present, notify the doctor. In rare cases, you may see signs of anaphylactic shock. Be prepared to administer epinephrine hydrochloride (Sus-Phrine*), as ordered. Notify the doctor if these signs appear.
    If patient complains of severe abdominal distention and pain with muscle guarding, and develops a fever suspect internal bleeding, bile peritonitis, or developing septicemia. Notify the doctor if he makes such a complaint.

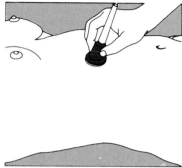

ULTRASOUND

Purpose
• Performed if patient has an iodine allergy, a liver disorder, gastric outlet obstruction, or if other tests prove unsuccessful.
• Patient's liver does not need to be functioning normally.
• Uses sound waves to detect gallstones or duct strictures.

Procedure
• Ultrasound transducer's slowly moved over lubricated abdominal surface.

Nursing preparations
• Withhold foods and oral fluids (except water) for 12 hours before test to prevent stomach distention.
• If patient's stomach is distended, be prepared to insert a nasogastric tube, as ordered.
• Administer simethicone (Mylicon), as ordered, to prevent gas and bloating.
• Do not allow barium studies performed prior to ultrasound testing. Barium reflects sound waves.

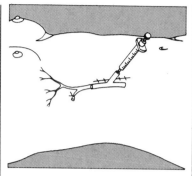

T TUBE CHOLANGIOGRAM

Purpose
• To determine common bile duct patency before T tube removal.

Procedure
• Contrast dye injected into T tube during X-ray procedure

Nursing preparations
• Obtain accurate history of patient's allergies, especially to seafood and iodine. Remember, the contrast dye used in this test contains iodine.
• Withhold foods and oral fluids for 10 to 12 hours before X-ray.
• Administer a sedative 1 hour before X-ray, as ordered.
• After the X-ray procedure, closely monitor patient for signs and symptoms of allergic reaction; for example, rash, diarrhea, and itching. If present, notify the doctor. In rare cases, you may see signs of anaphylactic shock. Be prepared to administer epinephrine hydrochloride (Sus-Phrine*), as ordered. Notify the doctor if these signs appear.

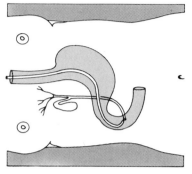

ENDOSCOPIC RETROGRADE
CHOLANGIOPANCREATOGRAPHY (ERCP)

Purpose
• Patient's liver does not need to be functioning normally to have this test.
• To visualize hepatic and pancreatic ducts, cystic and common bile duct, and gallbladder
• To diagnose the cause of jaundice, or to confirm suspected pancreatic diseases, common bile duct or gallbladder stones
• To detect and diagnose biliary system strictures, dilation, obstruction, or other abnormalities

Procedure
• Endoscope is passed orally into duodenum.
• Contrast dye is injected through endoscope into biliary tree.

Nursing preparations
• Obtain accurate history of patient's allergies, especially to iodine and seafood. Remember, the contrast dye used in this test contains iodine.
• Withhold foods and oral fluids for 8 hours before X-ray.
• Administer a sedative, as ordered, to ease endoscope insertion.
• Be prepared to assist doctor with endoscope insertion.
• Administer atropine sulfate or glucagon, as ordered, to relax duodenum and duct muscles.
• After the X-ray, closely monitor patient for signs and symptoms of allergic reaction; for example, rash, diarrhea, and itching. If present, notify the doctor. In rare cases, you may see signs of anaphylactic shock. Be prepared to administer epinephrine hydrochloride (Sus-Phrine*), as ordered. Notify the doctor if these signs appear. Also be alert for signs and symptoms of infection or chemical pancreatitis: fever, chills, abdominal tenderness, nausea, or vomiting. If present, notify the doctor.

*Available in both the United States and in Canada

Hepatic disorders

Knowing how to care for a patient with cirrhosis is one part of managing hepatic disorders. But are you familiar with the three types of hepatitis? Or how to care for a patient with a LeVeen shunt? Or, how to prepare a patient for a liver biopsy?

Whether your patient has hepatitis, ascites, or cirrhosis, the photos, illustrations, and guidelines in the next section will help you understand how to assess his condition and care for him. In addition, you'll also learn how to prepare a patient for abdominal paracentesis.

Read the following pages carefully.

Learning about hepatitis

Three basic types of hepatitis exist: A, B, and non-A/non-B. As you can see, all three types exhibit similar signs and symptoms. However, type non-A/non-B usually persists longer and may lead to chronic hepatitis.

What can you do for a patient with hepatitis? For starters, make sure he has adequate rest and proper nutrition. To help prevent mental depression and boredom, encourage him to read, work word puzzles, or participate in any other activity or hobby he can do in bed.

Keep in mind that your patient may be frightened or apprehensive about his hospital stay. Establish a rapport with your patient by encouraging him to talk about his feelings.

Also, devote some time to teaching your patient and his family about hepatitis, including how it's spread. Answer all of their questions. Then, be sure to document any patient teaching in your nurses' notes.

Type	Contamination sources	Incubation period	Signs and symptoms (prodromal)
A (Hepatitis A virus)	• Raw shellfish • Water • Oral contact with fecal matter • Blood and body secretions (in rare cases)	• 21 to 35 days; averages 30 days	• Mental and physical fatigue • Nausea; vomiting • Anorexia • Diarrhea • Right upper quadrant pain from liver distention • Headache • Hives or skin rash • Possible joint pain; arthritis in distal joints • Angioneurotic edema (edema of skin, mucous membranes, and occasionally viscera) • Elevated serum glutamic-oxaloacetic transaminase (SGOT) and serum glutamic-pyruvic transaminase (SGPT) levels 1 to 2 weeks prior to the appearance of jaundice • Flulike symptoms, including sore throat, cough, irritated nasal mucous membrane, and fever of 100° to 104° F. (37.8° to 40° C.)
B (Hepatitis B virus)	• Vaginal or anal intercourse • Breast milk • Syringes and needles • Saliva • Blood	• 60 to 150 days; averages 90 days	• Low grade fever of 100° to 101° F. (37.8° to 38.3° C.) • Mental and physical fatigue • Nausea; vomiting • Anorexia • Diarrhea • Right upper quadrant pain from liver distention • Headache • Hives or skin rash • Possible joint pain; arthritis in distal joints • Angioneurotic edema (edema of skin, mucous membranes, and occasionally viscera) • Elevated SGOT and SGPT levels 1 to 2 weeks prior to the appearance of jaundice • Symptoms worse than Type A • Diagnostic marker is presence of Hepatitis B Antigen (HBsAg), sometimes called Australian Antigen, in blood serum
NON A NON B (virus other than A or B)	• Blood transfusions • Syringes and needles	• 14 to 115 days; averages 50 days	• Mental and physical fatigue • Nausea; vomiting • Anorexia • Diarrhea • Right upper quadrant pain from liver distention • Headache • Hives or skin rash • Possible joint pain; arthritis in distal joints • Angioneurotic edema (edema of skin, mucous membranes, and occasionally viscera) • Elevated SGOT and SGPT levels 1 to 2 weeks prior to the appearance of jaundice

Signs and symptoms (icteric)	Indications of recovery
• Dark yellow urine, clay-colored stools, yellowish mucous membrane and sclerae (jaundice) • Swollen lymph nodes, tender on palpation • Weight loss (5 to 15 pounds) • Moderately enlarged liver, tender on palpation • Increased SGOT and SGPT levels • Slightly increased alkaline phosphatase • Prolonged prothrombin time • Mild leukocytosis • Bilirubinemia • Bilirubin in urine, increased urobilinogen (above 4 mcg/24 hours)	• Gradual decrease of all symptoms. Stools, urine, skin, and sclerae return to normal color. • Gradual return of normal lab values • Recovery phase begins 1 to 2 weeks after jaundice subsides and usually lasts from 2 to 6 weeks. • Return of appetite as patient begins to feel better
• Same as Type A (more severe); possibly leading to massive liver necrosis and failure; and death	• Same as Type A
• Same as Type A, except patient may not develop jaundice	• Same as Type A • Recovery may last for months or may deteriorate to chronic hepatitis.

Learning about a liver biopsy

As you know, the doctor will perform a liver biopsy when he wants to learn more about your patient's liver pathology. For example, if he suspects cancer, or cirrhosis, he needs to perform a biopsy to make, or confirm, a diagnosis. However, such a biopsy is contraindicated if your patient's uncooperative, or has any of the following conditions: severe extrahepatic cholestasis; blood clotting problems; vascular malignant tumors; hepatic angiomas; congested liver, resulting from heart failure; or a hydatid cyst.

Wondering how a liver biopsy is performed? The doctor will insert a Vim-Silverman or modified Menghini needle into your patient's right side, in either her eighth or ninth intercostal space. Then, he'll extract a liver tissue sample and withdraw the needle.

You're responsible for preparing your patient mentally and physically. To do this, explain the procedure. Warn her that during the biopsy, and for a few days afterward, she'll feel some discomfort at the biopsy site. But, assure her that she'll receive a sedative before the procedure to help her relax and reduce any discomfort.

Then, have your patient practice holding her breath for 5 to 10 seconds. Tell her she'll need to do this as the doctor inserts the needle. Holding her breath keeps her chest from moving (and her liver still), and prevents a pleural cavity or diaphragm puncture.

Before the biopsy, obtain a sample of your patient's blood for type and cross match. Then, make sure a unit of the proper type blood's on hold, in case a transfusion is necessary. Also, withhold all food and oral fluids for 6 hours before the test, to decrease blood congestion in her liver.

Immediately before the procedure, tuck a pillow under your patient's right shoulder and back, and expose her right side (see photo). The doctor will prep the area with Betadine scrub. Then, he'll place a sterile fenestrated drape over the area, as shown in the inset. Continue to reassure your patient during the procedure.

After the procedure, apply a pressure bandage to the biopsy site. Tell your patient to lie on her right side for 2 hours after the test to splint the puncture site. Then, keep her on bed rest for the next 22 hours, or as ordered. Label and send the liver tissue specimen to the lab for analysis. Also, closely monitor your patient's vital signs. If her blood pressure decreases, pulse rate increases, or if she complains of pain in her upper right quadrant (indicating hemorrhage or bile peritonitis), notify the doctor.

In addition, check the injection site every 30 minutes for the first 4 hours after the biopsy, then hourly for the next 8 hours. If you see bleeding or a hematoma at the site, notify the doctor.

Document the procedure in your notes.

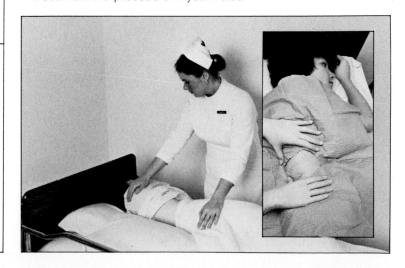

Hepatic disorders

Understanding liver cirrhosis

Caring for a patient with cirrhosis of the liver can be challenging. Why? Because the disease only becomes evident in the advanced stage. By this time, more than 50% of the liver has been destroyed, and can't regenerate. As cirrhosis progresses, the liver becomes hard, shrunken, and nodular (see illustration). Slowly, it loses its ability to function properly.

The early signs and symptoms of cirrhosis (such as change in bowel habits, lassitude, and dyspepsia) sometimes go unreported. But, the more advanced signs (anorexia, weight loss [which, incidentally, may be masked by fluid retention], ascites, peripheral edema, abdominal pain, and jaundice) cause alarm. Your ability to recognize and control these signs and symptoms is a major part of your nursing responsibility. Follow these guidelines to provide better care for your patient:
* Provide small, frequent meals that are high in carbohydrates and bulk. Encourage your patient to eat and try to give him a choice of foods.
* Orally administer supplementary vitamins A, B complex, and C, as ordered.
* Elevate the head of your patient's bed to ease his breathing and promote rest.
* Administer vitamin K, I.M. or orally, as ordered, to control bleeding. When giving I.M. injections, use a small-gauge needle. If bleeding results from the injection, document the location and amount. Then, notify the doctor.
* To prevent nausea and vomiting, administer antiemetics, I.M., as ordered. Give before meals, if possible.
* Whenever possible, encourage your patient to use the toilet instead of a bedpan, or provide a bedside commode.
* Provide cholestyramine (Questran*) orally; or cool baking-soda baths to relieve itching from jaundice, as ordered.
* To control edema, restrict sodium intake, and apply antiembolism stockings, if ordered.
* When your patient's seated in a chair, elevate his legs on a footstool, to prevent ankle edema.
* Document everything in your nurses' notes.

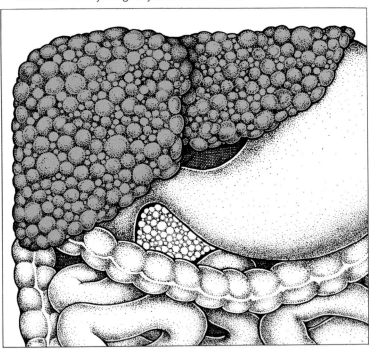

Understanding ascites

Does your patient have ascites? To find out, assess your patient's abdomen, as shown at right. Although ascites, the accumulation of fluid in the abdomen, may be caused by heart or renal failure, it's usually the result of cirrhosis. However, the pathophysiology is extremely complex and not completely understood.

But what causes the fluid to accumulate? Let's consider a patient with cirrhosis: veins in his liver are obstructed, elevating portal venous pressure. When portal venous pressure rises 3 to 5 mm Hg above normal, large amounts of fluid leak through the liver's surface into the abdominal cavity, causing ascites. In mild cases, the condition can be treated medically with diuretics and restricted fluid and sodium intake. However, sometimes the ascites is so advanced that it interferes with the patient's breathing. In such cases, the doctor may perform an abdominal paracentesis (see page 151), which will provide temporary relief until the underlying condition is controlled.

When the underlying problem can't be controlled—for example, with cirrhosis—the doctor may decide to surgically insert a LeVeen shunt (as described on page 152). When the shunt's in place, ascitic fluid is shunted from the abdominal cavity and reinfused into the venous system.

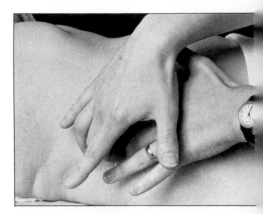

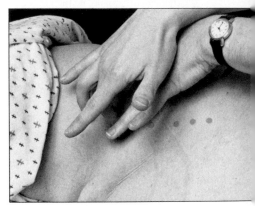

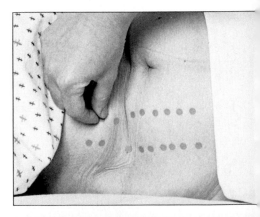

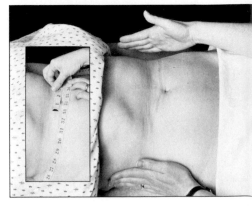

*Available in both the United States and in Canada

How to assess your patient for ascites

1 *Let's say your patient has a distended abdomen with disproportionately bulging flanks. You suspect ascites. So, continue to check her abdomen for other telltale signs of this condition: tight, glistening abdominal skin; prominent veins; and a protruding umbilicus. If you see any or all of these, use the following guidelines to confirm and evaluate her condition.*

First, explain the procedure to your patient and place her in a supine position. Expose her abdomen.

Starting at her iliac crest, percuss along her right flank until you reach her lowest rib. If you hear a dull sound as you percuss, suspect fluid in your patient's abdomen.

2 Now, returning to her iliac crest, percuss 2″ (5 cm) above the first line of percussion across her right flank. Then, percuss 2″ (5 cm) above this line. Continue percussing until you no longer hear a dull sound. Mark this area with stick-on dots or a felt-tip pen.

Repeat this entire procedure on your patient's left flank.

3 Next, help your patient turn onto her right side. Percuss her abdomen from her right flank upward toward her umbilicus. When you no longer hear a dull sound, stop percussing and mark this location, as the nurse is doing here. If your patient has ascites, the line of dullness will probably be near her midline.

4 Suppose your patient's abdomen is grossly distended. Then, perform the fluid wave test. To do this, place your patient on her back and put your left palm on her right flank. Firmly tap her left flank with your right hand, as shown here. Any large accumulation of fluid in her abdomen (advanced ascites) will cause a fluid wave to ripple across her abdomen. You'll feel this wave on her right flank.

[Inset] Now, measure and record your patient's abdominal girth. Measure her abdominal girth daily, preferably before breakfast. Note and record any changes.

In your nurses' notes, document the procedure and all findings.

Abdominal paracentesis: Your role

If your patient has ascites, one of the doctor's first steps will be to restrict your patient's sodium and fluid intake. Then, he'll probably order diuretics, such as chlorothiazide (Diuril*), triamterene (Dyrenium*), or furosemide (Lasix*), administered daily. These steps are relatively simple, effective ways of dealing with ascites.

Despite these measures, fluid may continue to accumulate in your patient's abdomen. In such a case, the doctor may decide to drain the ascitic fluid through a tube inserted into the patient's abdomen. This procedure, called abdominal paracentesis, temporarily relieves ascites.

In most cases, the doctor performs this procedure in the patient's room. You'll be expected to assist according to his instructions. Here's how:

First, instruct your patient to urinate. Then, if possible, seat him in a chair with his back well supported and his feet flat on the floor. (If your patient can't tolerate sitting in a chair, place him in a high Fowler's position in bed, as ordered.) Prep his abdomen with Betadine scrub, and stand by as the doctor uses a scalpel to make a small incision in the patient's abdomen. He'll then insert a trocar (a plastic cannula with a metal guide) into the incision. Next, he'll remove the metal guide, leaving the plastic cannula in place. In some cases, he may suture the cannula in place. The end of the cannula is then connected to a drainage tube.

Because most patients with ascites also have peripheral edema, the doctor usually allows 3 to 5 liters of ascitic fluid to flow into the drainage bag. In most cases, this takes 1 hour.

But, if the patient doesn't have peripheral edema, the doctor drains only enough fluid to relieve the patient's symptoms. This avoids pulling an excessive amount of fluid from the patient's vascular system and minimizes the risk of hypovolemic shock.

Of course, you should remain with your patient during the entire procedure. Be sure to record your patient's vital signs every 15 minutes, as the nurse is doing here. Stay alert for signs of shock: increased pulse rate, decreased blood pressure, and diaphoresis. If you see any of these signs, clamp the drainage tube with a hemostat. Then, help your patient into bed (if he isn't there already), and place him

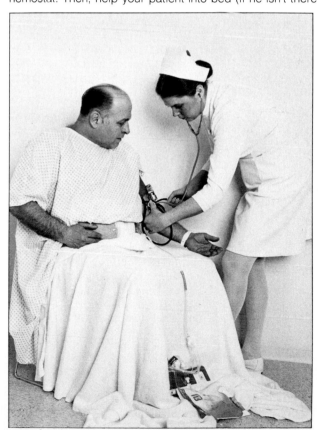

in a low Fowler's position. Notify the doctor.

After the prescribed amount of ascitic fluid has drained, record the amount, color, and consistency of the drainage. Also, record the drainage amount as output. Send specimens to the lab, as ordered. Then, remove the cannula (in some hospitals the doctor does this), and apply a sterile dressing to the incision site.

For the next 24 hours, monitor your patient's vital signs and check his dressing for drainage. If you see any drainage, change the dressing. Also, keep a daily record of his weight, abdominal girth, and urinary output.

Document the procedure.

*Available in both the United States and in Canada

Hepatic disorders

Caring for a patient with a LeVeen shunt

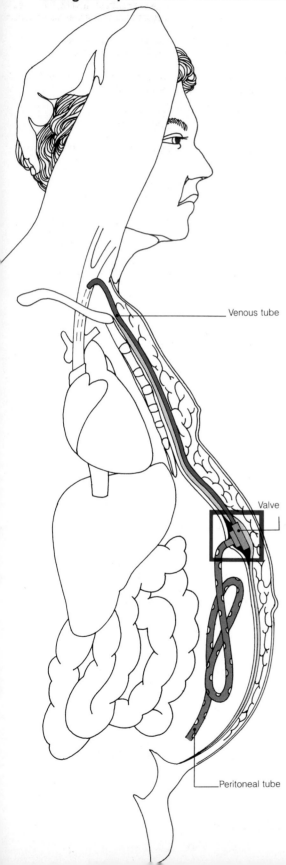

Venous tube

Valve

Peritoneal tube

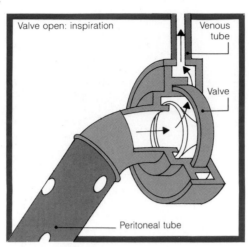

Valve open: inspiration

Venous tube

Valve

Peritoneal tube

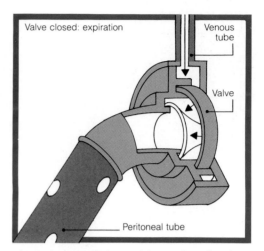

Valve closed: expiration

Venous tube

Valve

Peritoneal tube

If you've ever cared for a patient with intractable ascites, you may be familiar with the LeVeen shunt. But, most likely, you're not quite sure how it works.

When surgically inserted, a LeVeen shunt continuously reinfuses ascitic fluid into the patient's venous system. As shown in the illustration at left, the shunt consists of a peritoneal tube, a venous tube, and a one-way valve controlling fluid flow.

How does the shunt work? As your patient inhales, his abdominal pressure increases and superior vena cava pressure decreases. This pressure differential forces the valve open, allowing fluid to flow from the abdomen into the superior vena cava (above left). Then, as your patient exhales, his superior vena cava pressure increases and abdominal pressure decreases. This pressure differential causes the valve to close, stopping the fluid flow (above right).

But, suppose your patient develops congestive heart failure and his superior vena cava pressure remains greater than his abdominal pressure at all times. In this case, the shunt's valve stays shut—a built-in safety feature—reducing the danger of fluid overload in his vascular system. The valve also prevents blood from flowing back into the venous tube, blocking the shunt.

You'll be responsible for preparing your patient for LeVeen shunt surgery and caring for him after surgery. Begin by explaining what the shunt is and how it can help him. Also, take this opportunity to teach him how to breathe into a blow bottle. This breathing against resistance will help ascitic fluid flow more smoothly after the shunt's in place.

As part of your daily routine (before and after surgery): measure and record your patient's weight and abdominal girth; keep accurate intake and output records; send 24-hour urine specimens to the lab for

*Available in both the United States and in Canada

electrolyte analysis; and (as ordered) administer prophylactic antibiotic therapy. For 2 days immediately before and after surgery, the doctor'll want blood specimens sent to the lab for an SMA6, SMA12, and CBC. If the lab report shows a below-normal hematocrit level, be prepared to administer a blood transfusion, as ordered by the doctor. Also, be sure to check the lab results for your patient's potassium level. Notify the doctor if the level is below normal.

After your patient returns from surgery, try to make him as comfortable as possible. Place him in either a low or semi-Fowler's position, whichever he prefers. Put the blow bottle near his bed and remind him to use it 4 times a day, 15 minutes each time.

Next, as ordered, you'll administer 80 mg furosemide (Lasix*) I.M. or I.V. to reduce fluid retention. Keep an accurate hourly urine output record. If your patient's urine output decreases to 30 ml or less, be prepared to administer additional doses of furosemide, as ordered.

During the first 24 hours postop, you'll send blood specimens to the lab for hematocrit analysis every 4 hours. If the hematocrit level is below normal, notify the doctor.

About 24 to 48 hours after surgery, the doctor'll probably want your patient placed on a regular or sodium-restricted diet.

After 48 hours, you'll obtain blood specimens for SMA6, SMA12, and CBC every 2 to 3 days, as ordered.

Also, be alert for signs of possible complications, such as ascitic fluid leakage or infection at both incision sites, subcutaneous bleeding, disseminated intravascular coagulation (DIC), gastrointestinal bleeding, septicemia, shunt occlusion, and congestive heart failure.

Remember to document all procedures in your nurses' notes.

Pancreatic disorders

How familiar are you with pancreatic disorders? For example, do you know the signs and symptoms of acute pancreatitis? Or the difference between acute and chronic pancreatitis?

What about caring for the patient with pancreatic cancer? Do you know how to prepare him for Whipple's operation?

If you're not sure, pay special attention to the information that follows. You'll find the answers to these questions as well as additional information to help you sharpen your nursing skills.

Learning about pancreatitis

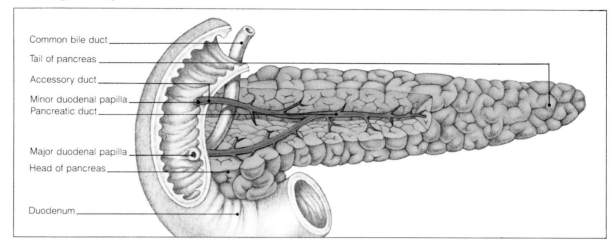

Common bile duct
Tail of pancreas
Accessory duct
Minor duodenal papilla
Pancreatic duct
Major duodenal papilla
Head of pancreas
Duodenum

Before you care for a patient with pancreatitis, review the information to the right.

As you may know, the signs and symptoms of acute pancreatitis develop quickly, and last only a short time.

First, the abdominal pain will disappear (usually within 48 hours), then the other signs and symptoms.

In many cases, the patient will never have another acute pancreatitis attack.

But, chronic pancreatitis recurs. Although the signs and symptoms of chronic pancreatitis develop more slowly, they usually last for 3 to 7 days. And, as the disease progresses, the intervals between attacks may become shorter until signs and symptoms are constant.

Keep in mind, however, that patients with chronic pancreatitis may be totally asymptomatic between attacks.

ACUTE PANCREATITIS

Possible causes
- Gallstones
- Chronic alcoholism
- Hyperlipidemia
- History of blunt or penetrating abdominal trauma
- Degenerative vascular disease
- Drug side effects from: chlorothiazides, isoniazid, salicylates, and immunosuppressants used to treat pancreatitis

Signs and symptoms
- Acute abdominal pain, especially in epigastric area. May radiate to back.
- Nausea and vomiting
- Low-grade fever: 100° to 102° F. (37.8° to 38.9° C.)
- Shock: tachycardia; cold, clammy skin; rapid pulse; decreased blood pressure
- Increased leukocyte level in blood (usually over 16,000 per cu mm)
- Ecchymosis around umbilicus (Cullen's sign), and on flanks (Turner's sign)
- Restlessness and anxiety
- Delirium tremens, if patient's an alcoholic
- Possible jaundice
- Possible abdominal distention
- Increased levels of serum amylase, serum lipase, serum glucose, and direct bilirubin

Nursing considerations
- Withhold food and fluids until acute symptoms (abdominal pain, vomiting, and nausea) subside.
- Insert a nasogastric (NG) tube, as ordered, to aspirate gastric contents, reduce nausea and vomiting, and prevent stimulation of pancreatic secretions.
- Place patient in knee-chest position or have him lean forward to relieve abdominal pain.
- Be prepared to administer analgesic drugs, as ordered, to help reduce pain. Avoid giving morphine sulfate and its derivatives, as they may cause spasms of the sphincter of Oddi.
- Administer anticholinergic drugs, as ordered, to help reduce GI motility.
- Administer antibiotic drugs, as ordered, to help reduce infection.
- Obtain blood specimens to determine serum electrolyte levels; complete blood count; serum amylase, serum lipase, serum glucose, and direct bilirubin levels.
- Insert a Foley catheter, as ordered. Keep accurate intake and output records
- Be alert for magnesium or calcium deficiencies; hyperactive tendon reflexes; seizures; and muscle tremors. If signs and symptoms are present, notify the doctor and be prepared to administer magnesium sulfate or calcium gluconate I.V.
- Give vitamins, as ordered, to supplement patient's diet.
- Watch for signs of hypo- or hyperglycemia. Give insulin or dextrose in water, as ordered.

Pancreatic disorders

Learning about pancreatitis continued

CHRONIC PANCREATITIS

Possible causes
- Chronic alcoholism
- Repeated attacks of acute pancreatitis
- Malnutrition

Signs and symptoms
During attack:
- Burning or gnawing abdominal pain, radiating to back, and aggravated by food or alcohol
- Nausea or vomiting
- Low grade fever: 100° to 102° F. (37.8° to 38.9° C.)
- Shock: tachycardia, cold, clammy skin, rapid pulse, decreased blood pressure
- Increased leukocyte level in blood (usually over 16,000 per cu mm)
- Ecchymosis around umbilicus (Cullen's sign) and on flanks (Turner's sign)
- Restlessness and anxiety
- Abdominal tenderness
- Delirium tremens, if patient's an alcoholic
- Possible jaundice
- Possible abdominal distention

Between attacks:
- May be asymptomatic
- Frequent, frothy, foul-smelling stools (steatorrhea), from impaired digestion of fatty foods
- Weight loss
- Possible jaundice
- Constant, vague abdominal discomfort, and epigastric fullness

Nursing considerations
- Provide frequent low-fat meals, high in carbohydrates and proteins. Instruct patient to completely avoid alcohol, and to limit excessive intake of caffeinic beverages.
- Administer analgesic drugs to relieve pain, as ordered. Avoid giving morphine sulfate and its derivatives, as they may cause spasms of the sphincter of Oddi.
- Give antacid and anticholinergic drugs, as ordered, to reduce GI motility.
- Administer digestant drugs, such as bile salts, pancreatin, and pancrelipase, as ordered, to aid digestion of fat, and help fat-soluble vitamin absorption.
- Be alert for signs of diabetes mellitus: polydipsia, polyuria, polyphagia, fruity breath, and dry, flushed skin. If you see these signs and symptoms, notify the doctor.

What you should know about Whipple's operation

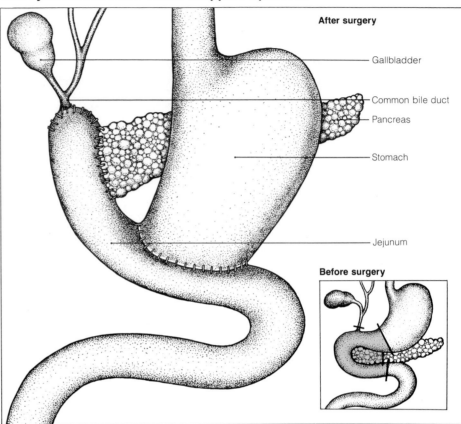

After surgery

Gallbladder

Common bile duct

Pancreas

Stomach

Jejunum

Before surgery

Caring for a patient with pancreatic cancer? If so, the doctor may decide to perform a pancreatoduodenectomy (Whipple's operation). As you probably know, this procedure involves removing the head of the pancreas and portions of its body and tail; the duodenum; portions of the stomach; the pancreatic duct; and the distal portion of the common bile ducts. (In some cases, the gallbladder may also be removed.) When that's accomplished, the remaining portions of the stomach, pancreas and common bile duct are anastomosed to the jejunum.

You'll begin preparing your patient 4 to 5 days before surgery. Because your patient's weak, you'll need to build up his strength. To do this, provide a low-fat diet high in carbohydrate and protein; give vitamin supplements orally; and administer 5% dextrose in water I.V., as ordered. The doctor may also want you to give vitamin K and blood transfusions.

Note: If your patient can't take food orally, the doctor may decide to feed him through a nasogastric (NG) tube or to provide total parenteral nutrition (TPN) through a central venous line.

When your patient returns to his room after surgery, be ready to attach his endotracheal tube (if he has one) to a respirator, and his NG tube to suction, as ordered. Make sure the flow rates of his central venous line and peripheral venous line are correct, and his T tube is draining properly. Then, as part of your routine postop procedure, monitor his vital signs and urine output; obtain blood specimens for lab analysis; and maintain NG tube patency. Stay alert for signs of renal failure, including oliguria or anuria with a decreased urine specific gravity, and increased serum blood urea nitrogen (BUN) and creatinine levels.

Try to keep your patient as comfortable as possible. Administer analgesic drugs to help relieve pain, as ordered. Be sure to change your patient's position at least every 2 hours to prevent pulmonary and vascular complications. Encourage him to deep breathe and cough.

In addition, watch for signs of possible complications, such as hemorrhage, infection, diabetes mellitus, and jaundice. If you see any, notify the doctor.

Document all procedures in your nurses' notes.

Acknowledgements

PATIENT PREPARATION

When your patient's scheduled for Whipple's operation

Let's consider the case of John Hanson, a 53-year-old mechanic with pancreatic cancer. After his subtotal gastrectomy 6 months ago, he thought he was back on the road to recovery. Now, he's returned to the hospital, scheduled for a pancreatoduodenectomy (Whipple's operation). The doctor has talked with him, but Mr. Hanson didn't understand what he was saying and was too nervous to ask questions. How can you help him?

As you know, preparing Mr. Hanson emotionally is a major part of your nursing responsibility. How do you feel about this? Do you find yourself avoiding a patient with cancer? Or pulling away emotionally? Maintaining control over your emotions is essential. But don't act remote. Because both cancer and radical surgery are frightening prospects, he probably needs a great deal of psychologic support.

When you first speak with Mr. Hanson, try to have members of his family present. Display anatomical illustrations of how the GI tract looks before and after surgery. The illustrations will help describe Whipple's operation. Then, clearly explain to your patient, and his family, that during surgery the doctor will remove parts of the stomach, pancreas, gallbladder duct, and small intestines. (In some cases, the gallbladder will also be removed.) Then, he'll connect the remaining portions of these organs together. Assure Mr. Hanson that he'll be able to return to his preoperative diet once he's recovered from surgery.

Encourage your patient and his family to ask questions. Answer them honestly, but don't give them false hope. If you're not sure how to answer, tell them you'll get the information.

After the initial session, try to talk to Mr. Hanson whenever possible, both before and after surgery. Because of the poor prognosis for pancreatic cancer, much of your nursing care will be supportive. Encourage him to talk about his disease, the surgery, his life, and, most important, his feelings. Listen to his concerns about himself and his family. Then, do your best to reassure him.

We'd like to thank the following people and companies for their help with this PHOTOBOOK:

AMERICAN PHARMASEAL
Glendale, Calif.
William Krieg, Product Manager, Nursing Services Products

C.R. BARD, INC.
Bard Urological Division
Murray Hill, N.J.

BIOSEARCH MEDICAL PRODUCTS INC.
Raritan, N.J.
Manfred F. Dyck, President

CHESEBROUGH-POND'S INC.
Hospital Products Division
Greenwich, Conn.

DAVOL INC.
Subsidiary of C.R. Bard, Inc.
Cranston, R.I.

HEALTHCO, INC.
Reading, Pa.
Al Szymborski, CMR

HEDECO
Mountain View, Calif.

HOLLISTER INCORPORATED
Libertyville, Ill.

IMED CORPORATION
San Diego, Calif.

MASON LABORATORIES, INC.
Horsham, Pa.
James H. Mason, President
John L. Waters, Exec. Vice-President

NATIONAL CATHETER CO.
Argyle, N.Y.
J. Thomas Burns, Director of Marketing

NU-HOPE LABORATORIES, INC.
Los Angeles, Calif.
Eugene Galindo, President

PROCTER & GAMBLE COMPANY
Patient Care Products Division
Cincinnati, Ohio

RUSCH INC.
New York, N.Y.

E.R. SQUIBB & SONS, INC.
Princeton, N.J.
James P. Capasso, Product Manager

SWEEN CORPORATION
Mankato, Minn.
Al Sween, President

Also the staff of:

QUAKERTOWN HOSPITAL
Quakertown, Pa.

Selected references

Books

ASSESSING YOUR PATIENTS. Nursing Photobook™ Series. Horsham, Pa.: Intermed Communications, Inc., 1981.

Berci, George, ed. ENDOSCOPY. New York: Appleton-Century-Crofts, 1976.

Beyers, Marjorie, and Susan Dudas. THE CLINICAL PRACTICE OF MEDICAL-SURGICAL NURSING. Boston: Little, Brown & Co., 1977.

Boyce, H. Worth, and Eddy D. Palmer. TECHNIQUES OF CLINICAL GASTROENTEROLOGY. Springfield, Ill.: Charles C. Thomas, Publishers, 1975.

Brunner, Lillian S., and Doris S. Suddarth. TEXTBOOK OF MEDICAL-SURGICAL NURSING, 4th ed. New York: J.B. Lippincott Co., 1980.

Cassileth, Barrie R. THE CANCER PATIENT: SOCIAL & MEDICAL ASPECTS OF CARE. Philadelphia: Lea & Febiger, 1979.

DEALING WITH EMERGENCIES. Nursing Photobook™ Series. Horsham, Pa.: Intermed Communications, Inc., 1978.

Fisher, Alexander A. CONTACT DERMATITIS, 2nd ed. Philadelphia: Lea & Febiger, 1973.

Given, Barbara A., and Sandra J. Simmons. GASTROENTEROLOGY IN CLINICAL NURSING. St. Louis: C.V. Mosby Co., 1979.

GIVING MEDICATIONS. Nursing Photobook™ Series. Horsham, Pa.: Intermed Communications, Inc., 1980.

Guyton, Arthur C. TEXTBOOK OF MEDICAL PHYSIOLOGY, 5th ed. Philadelphia: W.B. Saunders Co., 1976.

HELPING CANCER PATIENTS EFFECTIVELY. Nursing Skillbook® Series. Horsham, Pa.: Intermed Communications, Inc., 1978.

Henderson, Virginia. THE NITE GHADYS PRINCIPLES AND PRACTICE OF NURSING, 6th ed. New York: Macmillan Publishing Co., Inc., 1978.

Kirsner, Joseph B., and Roy G. Shorter, eds. INFLAMMATORY BOWEL DISEASE. Philadelphia: Lea & Febiger, 1975.

Knoben, James E., et. al. HANDBOOK OF CLINICAL DRUG DATA, 3rd ed. Hamilton, Ill.: Drug Intelligence Publications, 1973.

Luckmann, Joan, and Karen C. Sorensen. MEDICAL-SURGICAL NURSING: A PSYCHOPHYSIOLOGIC APPROACH, 2nd ed. Philadelphia: W.B. Saunders Co., 1980.

MacLeod, John, ed. DAVIDSON'S PRINCIPLES AND PRACTICE OF MEDICINE, 12th ed. London: Churchill Livingstone, Inc., 1978.

Mahoney, Joanne M. GUIDE TO OSTOMY NURSING CARE. Boston: Little, Brown & Co., 1976.

MANAGING I.V. THERAPY. Nursing Photobook™ Series. Horsham, Pa.: Intermed Communications, Inc., 1980.

May, Harriet J. ENTEROSTOMAL THERAPY. New York: Raven Press Publishers, 1977.

MONITORING FLUID AND ELECTROLYTES PRECISELY. Nursing Skillbook® Series. Horsham, Pa.: Intermed Communications, Inc., 1978.

NURSING CRITICALLY ILL PATIENTS CONFIDENTLY. Nursing Skillbook® Series. Horsham, Pa.: Intermed Communications, Inc., 1979.

Price, Sylvia and Lorraine Wilson. PATHOPHYSIOLOGY: CLINICAL CONCEPTS OF DISEASE PROCESSES. New York: McGraw-Hill Book Co., 1978.

PROVIDING RESPIRATORY CARE. Nursing Photobook™ Series. Horsham, Pa.: Intermed Communications, Inc., 1979.

Russo, Barbara A. GASTROENTEROLOGY NURSING—CONTINUING EDUCATION REVIEW. Garden City, N.Y.: Medical Examination Publishing Co., Inc., 1976.

Vokovich, Virginia C., and Reba G. Grubb. CARE OF THE OSTOMY PATIENT, 2nd ed. St. Louis: C.V. Mosby Co., 1977.

Zander, Karen S., and Kathleen A. Bower, eds. A PRACTICAL MANUAL FOR PATIENT-TEACHING. St. Louis: C.V. Mosby Co., 1978.

Periodicals

Baab, Richard R. *Diagnosis: Cause of ascites,* HOSPITAL MEDICINE. 43-50, December 1980.

Dicken, A. *Why patients should plan their own recovery,* RN. 41:52-5, March 1978.

From MI scare to total gastrectomy—in one incredible patient, RN. 41:63-9, October 1978.

Gendron, Diana. *Show me,* THE CANADIAN NURSE. 74:10-13, December 1978.

Griggs, Barbara A., and Mary C. Hoppe. *Update: Nasogastric tube feedings,* AMERICAN JOURNAL OF NURSING. 79:481-85, March 1979.

Is it gallbladder disease or isn't it? PATIENT CARE. 14:14-23, July 15, 1980.

Kratzer, Joan B. *What does your patient need to know?* NURSING77. 7:82-4, December 1977.

Long, Gail D'Onofrio. *G.I. bleeding: What to do and when,* NURSING78. 8:44-50, March 1978.

Penn, Israel. *Management of the perforated duodenal ulcer,* HEART & LUNG. 7:111-17, January-February 1978.

Volden, Cecilia, Jacquelyn Grinde, and David Carl. *Taking the trauma out of nasogastric intubation,* NURSING80. 10:64-7, September 1980.

Williamson, K. and N. McCray. *Putting together a patient education program that works,* RN. 40:53-5, November 1977.

Selected references for the patient with a GI disorder

Available from the American Cancer Society, Inc., 777 Third Ave., New York, NY 10017:
A NO-NONSENSE LOOK AT WHAT MAY BE THE MOST IMPORTANT DAYS OF YOUR LIFE!
THE MOST IMPORTANT WEEKS OF YOUR LIFE!
WHAT IS CHEMOTHERAPY?

Available from Metropolitan Life Insurance Company:
ALCOHOL AND HEALTH

Available from Ross Laboratories, Columbus, OH 43216:
NUTRITION: A HELPFUL ALLY IN CANCER THERAPY

Available from the United Ostomy Association, Inc., 1111 Wilshire Blvd., Los Angeles, CA 90017:
A VERY PRIVATE MATTER
ILEOSTOMY: A GUIDE
SEX AND THE MALE OSTOMATE
SEX, COURTSHIP AND THE SINGLE OSTOMATE
SEX, PREGNANCY AND THE FEMALE OSTOMATE
SO YOU HAVE—OR WILL HAVE AN OSTOMY

Available from the United States Department of Health, Education, and Welfare, Washington, DC 20203:
DIET AND NUTRITION. Publication No. 80-2038
EATING HINTS, RECIPES AND TIPS FOR BETTER NUTRITION DURING TREATMENT. Publication No. 80-2079
EVERYTHING DOESN'T CAUSE CANCER. Publication No. 80-2039
TREATING CANCER. Publication No. 77-210

Index

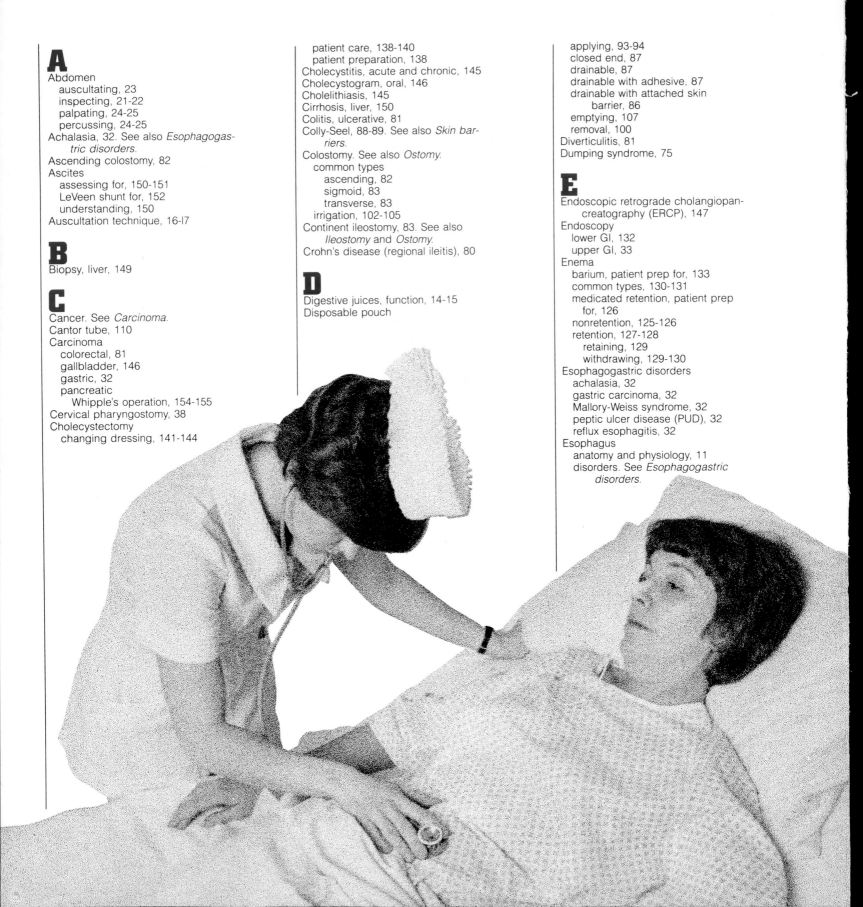

Index

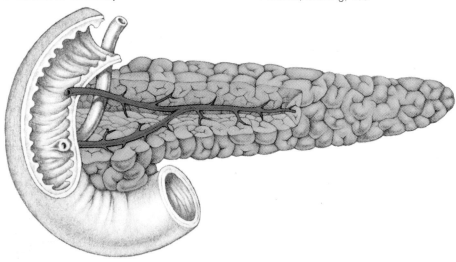